51 Ways
to Pick Up
Your
Get-Up-and-Go

To Judith,
You have a special
spirit! Thank-you!

Shauna Schlick
5/02

51 Ways
to Pick Up
Your
Get-Up-and-Go

Shawna Schuh

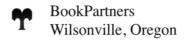
BookPartners
Wilsonville, Oregon

Copyright 1999 by Shawna Schuh
All rights reserved
Printed in U.S.A.
Library of Congress Catalog 98-74293
ISBN 1-58151-022-5

Cover design by Richard Ferguson
Text design by Sheryl Mehary

BookPartners, Inc.
P. O. Box 922
Wilsonville, Oregon 97071

This book is dedicated to
Gil and Louise Schuh, my loving,
giving, incredible parents
who loved me enough to teach me to
get up and go.
They're a wonderful pair of Schuhs!

Contents

Acknowledgments

51 and counting…
The following stories and the pickups that follow them are a tiny part of the intricate framework that makes up my life and continues to allow me to develop into the human being God intended me to be. I feel blessed and grateful that each day I have the opportunity to get up and get going all over again. I also feel blessed to have many people who help me.

My soul mate and husband, Don Potesta, is my supporter, prodder, cheerleader and sounding board. His love and support during this process is the only way I could have gotten this firstborn book pushed out of me. Thank you, Don, I love my life with you.

My fabulous friends are a constant avenue of strength, love and good common sense, especially Marianne Doherty, Rose Milbeck and Patsy Freeman who spent many hours helping me through this process. The others who have been a strong inspiration and given me motivation are too numerous to list but I'm sure they know who they are and how much I love them.

I would also like to thank Thorn Bacon, who took time to listen to my stories, read them, edit them and believe in them.

My hope for this book is that it will make you think, remember and take action. Each story we live, tell about and share brings us one step closer to being more fully alive. What's remarkable to me is that all of us have similar stories and ways in which we deal with the world. These stories are my way of sharing something I'm continuing to learn: We know the answers if we stop and think, listen and do.

1

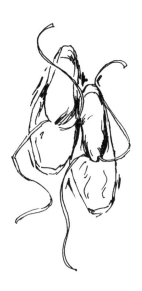

Dance to Your Own Beat

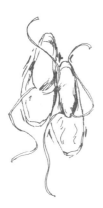

Dance to Your Own Beat

There is the greatest practical benefit in making a few failures early in life.

—T. H. Huxley

When Mom signed me up for dance lessons at the ripe old age of five I had no clue what I was doing, so I went with the flow and the ballet master's instructions: "Point your toe and put it back, take a step to the side, put your arms above your head and smile."

We all wore short-sleeved, royal blue leotards with a scooped neck, powder-pink tights with an uncomfortable seam up the back and powder-pink ballet shoes. Each girl's hair had to be pulled back into a bun and you weren't allowed to talk.

I endured it on beautiful fall afternoons while my brother and his friends got to play outside. The lessons were going to help me be graceful and ladylike, my mother told me. Whatever.

Crouched down in the back seat of the car, I changed into my dance outfit while Mom drove me all the way from our house in Helvetia, into Beaverton, where the dance school was located. The studio was tucked away in a single-story building with a wide royal blue door and a brass doorknob. Thick, royal-blue pile carpet in the waiting room muffled scurrying feet. The two classrooms had hardwood floors, and wooden double bars were mounted on three of the walls for warm-up exercises. Floor-to-ceiling mirrors dominated the fourth wall. Down a long hall, next to a big room smelling of sweat, used leather shoes and hair spray, were the dressing room and bathroom. I didn't often venture into the dressing room, because the big girls hung out there between classes.

At five years of age, I didn't see the point in taking lessons. Ballet was my mom's idea. I didn't want to point my toe in the company of other girls—little strangers who made faces at me after class. But I was swept along by the river of my mother's passion, which was swift, strong and undeniable.

For Christmas that year I got a new ballet case made of shiny black patent leather, with pictures of ballerinas on the front and a place to keep my ballet slippers inside. Kevin, my older brother, made fun of it: "Aren't we the little dancer!" he taunted me. "Little Miss Bun Head has a brand new bag." I began to hate dance lessons.

I didn't want to go each week and stumble around. This wasn't my idea of fun. But Mom wasn't going to give up on her dream of having an adorable little ballerina in the family. So, for the next five years, I went to ballet class every week and muddled through. I'd like to say I got a lot better during those years, and that my incredible dancing talent became obvious as time went on. Unfortunately, I seemed to get worse with each passing year. When I reached that indeterminate age just before puberty, when my baby fat and freckles defined me as too old for cute and too young to be noticed, I became an embarrassment to my mother.

I didn't want to go to ballet class, I didn't apply myself and I didn't care. I had absolutely no vision of myself dancing gracefully across the floor. Instead, I proved the old adage that you can't make a silk purse out of a sow's ear—which was one of my mother's favorite expressions.

Then one day, as we were rehearsing a recital dance, the teacher handed out the most wonderful cheerleader-type pompoms for us to hold in our arms. I was ecstatic! Suddenly, the whole class took on a new color and brightness. Pompoms seemed very grown up to my seven-year-old mind. Secretly, I had always wanted to be a cheerleader, which was much more in keeping with my budding personality. I wanted to yell! I wanted to jump and bounce and shout and scream. I wanted to be right in the action, with my hair flowing and my adrenaline pounding. Instead, I was stuck dancing classical ballet with my hair in a bun.

Our ballet master encouraged us to make some pompoms at home for practice, and I couldn't wait to leave class to begin this wonderful project. The pompoms idea gave me hope for something more vibrant than the endless drone of classical piano music and structured movements that made up my weekly ballet class.

"Remember you should make them yourself!" she shouted out to us as we scurried off to our mothers, who were patiently waiting in the lobby area.

"Oh, Mom! Guess what? Guess what?" I jumped up and down with excitement. Mom was fabulously calm and gave me her whole attention. "We're going to use pompoms in our dance and the teacher told us to make some for practice so we have to go buy stuff right now!" I threw in a few more tiny hops to make my point.

"OK, Shawna! Isn't that exciting?" She was caught up in my enthusiasm; finally I was showing a little initiative.

I vividly remember the red and white crepe paper I painstakingly picked out. I enlisted my brother, who was very good at art, to help me cut the long strips necessary to make the big balls of color. But things didn't turn out quite like I had envisioned. The scissors got stuck a lot and I wasn't very good at cutting straight, and I absolutely refused to let Kevin take over, no matter how hard he tried to persuade me. "No! I'm supposed to do it myself!" I wailed as I dripped glue everywhere, which soaked through the crinkly paper and stuck to about a bazillion other strips to form a large, clod-like knob on my wilting pompoms. "They'll look better after they dry," I tried to console myself.

"Sure they will!" Kevin assured me. I should have known better than to trust anything he said.

The next day they looked worse and there was no time to redo them. The only consolation I had was that I had truly done them all myself, which is exactly what the teacher had said to do. Also, those red and white pompoms could set me apart from the rest of my class. I hated that all of us dressed exactly alike, but at seven years of age, what are ya gonna do?

I was proud that I had followed the rules to the letter in making my pompoms, even though I wasn't proud of the product. In retrospect, it's sad that the only thing about my experience I was proud of was a set of disfigured and dissolving pompoms.

Before the next class, each girl sat in the waiting area with her pompoms on her lap. The inevitable comparisons began immediately. One very pretty, petite little blonde girl had the most incredible purple and silver pompoms you've ever seen. The purple was deep and vibrant, and the silver was shiny mylar. Her pompoms were full and round, just like the picture our teacher had shown us. The other dancers and I gathered around this little girl and she told us how her mother had had them made special just for her.

Well, that did it for me; I lifted my chin and announced quite loudly, "I did what the teacher said and made mine myself!" Self-righteousness dripped from my voice.

She took one look at my pompoms and said with disdain, "It looks like it."

I felt as though a ton of bricks falling on my head would not have crushed me as badly as her words. If the earth had opened up and swallowed me it would have been fine, I thought. The other girls looked at me and my wilty pompoms in disgust and turned their backs until class started. After that comment, the hardest thing for me to do was to carry those pompoms, but somehow I did. I didn't want to. I wanted to run and throw them into the trash and never go back to that class. But back I went, week after week, glumly gripping those hideous pompoms. Even after I told my mom what had happened and begged her not to make me use them or return to class, she persisted. "If you can't face up to things now, what kind of a person will you be?"

Right then I really didn't care, but I learned a pretty good lesson: Sometimes you must be prodded to get up and get going. Now, I thank my mom for making me finish the class with those pompoms. It was painful, but I learned that I was still me even after someone ridiculed me or made fun of what I created.

Looking back at that episode I can smile, because the weekly classes and all those agonizing hours at the ballet barre taught me the hard lesson of flow. Flow is about continuousness, the ever powerful movement of the universe onward, whether you're ready to go along or not. Flow means getting up and getting going even when you don't want to; even after you've been put down, stomped on or ridiculed. But I didn't understand flow when I was seven years old. The only message I heard in the little blonde girl's comment—which exemplified my entire ballet experience—was "you're not good enough." Fortunately, as I grew up I learned to add the word *yet* to the end of that sentence. You're not good enough yet. I now realize that no matter what endeavor I undertake, at first I will probably not be good enough. But that's what flow is all about. If I keep going, if I stay in the flow, eventually I will be good enough. We all will—it's a matter of time and doing what your heart calls you to.

Over the next couple of years, I discovered that something exciting was going on at the dance school, and it began to spark an interest in me. In the other room across the hall the older girls were hanging out along the barre that encircled their room. From the beginning, the double wooden bars had been my nightmare as I clung with one hand and tried to find my balance to do my pliés and relevés. Now the barre was being used by girls dressed in an array of wonderful leotard colors and styles. Even better, every one of those girls had her hair down. I discovered they were enrolled in a jazz dance class. They seemed so sophisticated, and what they were doing looked like so much fun.

I peeked into the room just as the teacher put on some music that pulsed and thumped with a wonderful rhythm and beat. I watched, enthralled, as the girls began to move to the music, swiveling their shoulders and hips. I felt the music enter my soul and I suddenly wanted to dance! But Mom pulled me out of there and we drove home in silence until she said, "You certainly aren't applying yourself, Shawna." What could I say to that? She was right on the money.

"I had such high hopes for you, honey; don't you want to be a ballerina and wear those pretty tutus?"

She asked me the same question every year at recital time when I wriggled into a satin-and-net tutu, which itched and scratched and stuck out from my body like a foofy inner tube. I couldn't sit down or stand close to anyone without crushing my netted skirt and getting in trouble with Mom. We have pictures that document this torture, and of course I have a hideous grin on my face in every one.

"I think the jazz class looks fun," I said nonchalantly to her in the silence following her last question. "Well, you can put that idea out of your mind. You have to be thirteen to take jazz and that's nothing like the beautiful ballet!" She was right—and that's why I liked it! But she was also right that I wasn't old enough, yet, so I continued with ballet.

That year at the recital, for the first time Mom let me stay until the end of the performance, which allowed me to watch the big girls from the jazz class perform. They did a routine to "These Boots Are Made for Walking." It was unbelievable! The older girls also danced a fun and crazy ballet called "Hoe Down," complete with stomping and hollering and boys carrying the girls off the stage. Stomping and hollering and dancing—what great fun. Sign me up! I was entranced and engaged and couldn't wait to dance like that!

Alas, I was only ten and you couldn't take jazz or modern dance until you were thirteen. It seemed so unfair that these other girls got to dance and move and shout and have fun while I was stuck with piano music and the endless structured movements of ballet.

Now that I knew there was an alternative, my aversion to my lessons grew. Mom finally gave in and pulled me out of the ballet class. I still remember her words: "I'm not going to pay for something if you aren't going to practice and apply yourself. Someday you'll probably regret that you didn't continue on with this!"

My heart soared! My hair was free from the bun! The royal blue leotard was retired and I didn't have to endure ridicule a moment longer.

Jazz dancing became my dream—doing the Hoe Down, wearing the colorful costumes, feeling the music and the movement and the beat. I was passionate about dancing. I waited three years until the summer before I turned thirteen.

"Could I please take jazz this fall?" I asked one day when we were shopping. Her reply was swift, "Do you really think I would pay for dance lessons after you wasted all that time and money before?"

This could be a tougher sell than I thought.

"That's because it was ballet and I hate ballet." Twelve-year-olds are not the best with logic, but they make up for it in persistence. "I really, really, really want to take jazz, Mom…Pleeeasssssse!"

"We'll think about it," she said and I began to hope. Ever since my last recital, three years earlier, I had envisioned myself onstage doing the routines with the big girls. Becoming somebody special. Three years is a long time to dream about something and I was determined to try.

When I arrived for my first jazz class that fall, I was disappointed when I ended up back in the small ballet room and not, as I had hoped, with the older jazz group. The class in the big room was for all the girls who hadn't given up dance and were ready for more advanced moves. Nevertheless, I was in a jazz class and I was loving my hour once a week learning to move my hips and torso and each shoulder independently. I was good, too! At least I thought I was. Instead of being the worst dancer in the class, I looked around and figured that, for once, I was one of the best. Unfortunately, I began to act a little like those girls I had once despised and I looked down with pity at the girls who were slightly overweight and couldn't pick up the steps.

During my three-year hiatus when I'd been relieved of ballet, something amazing had happened to my body. I had lost the baby fat and even had a waist! I was suddenly as coordinated as Mom always said I was, and the jazz moves came so easily! When the music started, I felt wonderful and alive, and my body moved in the most interesting ways! Wow! I was finally in! I had found something I loved, something I was passionate about.

I felt sorry for the girls who just didn't get it. It never occurred to me that they might have been forced into my jazz class in the same way I had been forced to take ballet. It never dawned on me that I was acting like a snob toward them.

As the year progressed, I worked very hard at everything the instructor taught us and I practiced every day. I couldn't dance or practice enough. I loved all of it. I was living and doing exactly what I was called to do.

When it came time to place the class members in position for the recital, I was very excited. I knew I would probably be featured in the front row, dead center. I was the best dancer, after all, and front and center is where the best always danced.

We lined up against the back wall and the instructor took each girl by the hand and led her to an exact location. She took the girl whom I considered my closest competitor and placed her in the front row, a little off of center. I smiled. I knew then that we'd probably share center stage. Next, she placed one of the other talented girls in the spot I thought I would get. I had a twinge of uneasiness until I realized that the exact center would be in the second row, in the window made by the first row of girls. I smiled inwardly. Center after all, I thought. The teacher then placed a girl very carefully in each window in the second row, including the center position, while I continued to stand in the back against the barre.

I looked on in horror as the instructor placed every other girl in a designated spot. As each successive spot was filled, I assured myself that the next position would be mine. My self-righteous attitude had melted completely and fear was setting in. When the last girl was set on the end of the third row, leaving me standing at the barre alone, I didn't know what to do.

A sickening realization came over me that not only was I not the best dancer as I so smugly had assumed, I wasn't even good enough for the teacher to remember to place me. Old feelings of rejection and unworthiness, of not being good enough, began to overtake me. The instructor walked over to the phonograph to put on our music and I saw the other girls' faces reflected in the mirror. They sneered at me as if to say, "Serves you right for being so high and mighty all these months!"

I didn't know what to do but it was suddenly very important to me to dance. In those agonizing moments standing in the back alone, I realized I didn't care where I stood, or what place I had, I just wanted desperately to dance in this number that I had worked so hard to perfect. This feeling was new but gave me courage.

I cleared my throat. "Miss Gail?" My voice was just enough above a whisper that she was able to hear me. She stopped her hand in mid-air as it was descending to place the record on the turntable. She glanced over her shoulder at me. "Yes?" she said.

Yes? I was hoping she'd look over in horror at her mistake, apologize, and move me to a spot, any spot. Now what would I do? My voice came floating up from somewhere and I managed to squeeze out, "Um...you forgot me." I didn't want to show disrespect, even though I could feel the tears starting to well up in my eyes. Please don't cry, I thought to myself, please, please don't cry. All eyes were on her or me and I thought I might die any second.

"Oh," she said with a wave of her hand, "You're going to do a little solo at the beginning." With those words, she changed my life.

There were no triumphant looks from me to the others, no sudden burst of pride or exuberance. Instead, I felt incredibly grateful—grateful to dance, to perform, to have learned all that I had. Those few moments of utter despair, when I thought I wouldn't dance at all, shifted my perspective to such an extent that I have never been the same since.

Had I been placed in the center front, where I thought I belonged, and lorded it over the other girls, I might never have learned the lesson of grace. How grateful I am to Miss Gail, and God, for the learning experience of that class. The fact that I had worked hard didn't guarantee me anything. We are never guaranteed anything except that life will continue to flow swiftly, as long as we live and beyond. The flow will either move us along or drown us, depending on our ability to alter our minds.

I now spend time enjoying the flow. Each day, I bend into what comes my way rather than worry about what will be. I am still enthralled with and passionate about dance — but the dance is now called life. The beat and rhythm of living are exciting, ever changing and pulsing with possibilities. I can express myself without reservation, no matter where I'm placed in life, because of the wonderful, incredible opportunity I have — to dance.

Pickup #1:   Follow your own dream.

Going to ballet class because my mother thought it was wonderful turned out to be a fiasco. The more Mother pushed her dreams on me, the more I knew I couldn't comply. You must search in your heart for the thing you dream of doing. Only then will the motivation come and no one will need to prod you; you'll be proud to pursue your goal.

Pickup #2:   Dance to the music that moves you.

When I heard hard-driving dance music I realized that the desire to move was in me. Keep your ears and your heart open to find your kind of music and to enable yourself to move toward the things that you are called to.

Pickup #3:   Stay humble.

I'm glad that my dance instructor knocked me down a peg or two by not placing me in the front row or telling me too soon that I would solo. It taught me humility and although

I hurt at the time, the lesson has stuck with me ever since. Whenever we place ourselves above others we lose our sure footing. Pride goeth before a fall. Humility will not only keep you moving forward, but will interest others in helping you also.

So...

Follow your own dream.

Dance to the music that moves you.

Stay humble.

2

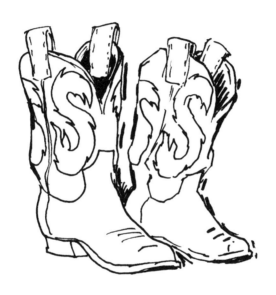

Do All You Can Do

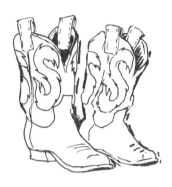

Do All
You Can Do

Where the willingness is great, the difficulties
cannot be great.

—Niccolo Machiavelli

"I can't do it, Daddy," I sobbed, with big, sloppy teardrops running down my face and nose.

"I can't get Wilbur to go!" I made my complaint in a high-pitched wail, which brought my dad forward in his lounge chair on the front porch. It was mid-July in Oregon and unseasonably hot. We lived in the country at Helvetia, an area known for its rolling hills, beautiful foliage and dairy farms. The grass in the front yard where my dad was stretched out was already dead and dry and looked like the yellow straw we used for bedding in the barn. I was at the end of my rope; I had tried everything to get my 4-H calf to move and lead and he wouldn't do it. He wouldn't follow my orders. I was failing. Worse yet, I knew the rules and I was breaking them.

I looked up at my dad through tear-filled eyes and waited for his verdict. When I had begged and pleaded with

Mom and Dad for a calf as a 4-H project, they had refused immediately. "You won't take care of it," they said. " It's too big of a project."

I could still hear their warnings: "Do you have any idea what having a baby calf will be like? You'll have to feed it morning and night, you'll have to clean its stall and make sure it's taken care of."

None of this mattered to me, because I had the cow bug so bad I couldn't see straight. I had just spent a week at the Washington County fair with my friend Teresa, whose family had a dairy farm nearby, and I had watched in wonder as kids just like me cleaned and cared for their animals. All shapes and sizes and ages of beautiful black and white Holsteins. I imagined myself in the show ring holding onto the biggest and best animal at the fair. I could smell the fresh, clean straw in my nose and feel the animal's short, coarse hair under my hands.

I pleaded with them for weeks until they relented, on the condition that I would buy the calf myself and I would be its total caretaker—no one else in the family would have to help me. The day they gave me permission was exciting and filled with anticipation. I was going to buy my very own calf.

I remember carefully counting out my hard-earned strawberry-picking money for Dad to take to the dairy farm. Forty dollars was the most money I had ever held in my hands and I took great pains in counting it. "Thirty-seven, thirty-eight, thirty-nine…" I was almost to the end, and as I placed the last dollar bill into Dad's massive hand, I knew I had made the right decision. I could hardly wait for him to get back from the farm.

Dad had convinced me to buy a bull calf, because most dairy farms were anxious to part with them for less money and I could eventually sell my calf at the auction and make a profit. I didn't care, I just wanted to love a calf and train it and go to the fair like my friend Teresa.

When Dad brought the trailer home there were two calves in it. I looked up in shock, "Why two, Daddy?" I only needed one, a perfect one.

"Well, I figured having an extra one would make yours eat better because of the competition, and then we can have one for the freezer when you sell yours."

His explanation made sense to me. I peeked over the trailer gate and my eyes rested on two baby calves standing side by side with their hind ends facing my way, a tall one that was mostly black and a smaller one that was mostly white.

"Wow, Daddy, which one's mine?" I asked in awe at this change of plans.

"You get to pick, sweetie," he said. I never imagined that I would have a choice. I had anticipated that Dad would bring only one animal home, which would be the perfect one. Now I had to choose. I took a long look at both of the calves. The tall one was very handsome and had a lot of black areas on his hide and four white legs, but he seemed a bit too perfect, a bit too assured. I glanced over at the little one, whose head was down as if he were frightened and didn't know what was going on. He looked as though he thought no one would want him, and when he glanced my way, I saw deep brown pools of fear staring back at me from the most adorable face, with a slobbery pink nose and long, white hairs sticking out of his chin.

"I want this one, Daddy," I said as I placed my hand on the white calf's scrawny, bony back.

My dad acted surprised. "But, honey," he said to me very gently, "Don't you think this other one is bigger and might do better at the fair?"

The fair had completely left my mind; all I could think was how this little calf that looked so small and scared needed me more than the other. I could help this one, but the other, self-sufficient one seemed not to need me at all.

"No, Daddy, this is the one," I said with even more determination. Dad then proceeded to point out all the deficiencies of my chosen calf. He was the same age as the other but only two-thirds the size; he was scrawny and a little malformed, his coat was mostly white, which was harder to keep clean; and he didn't look or act as healthy as his bigger companion.

"That's why he needs me," I replied, and that was the end of it. He was mine and I named him Wilbur.

Now, here I was, crying in front of my dad, a failure, unable to do what I so desperately wanted to do, which was to get my half-grown steer to lead for the show ring.

My dad took my chin in his hand and looked me in the eye. "Have you really tried, Shawna?" he asked. My dad stands six feet two and works in construction. He is big and muscular, with jet black hair that at the time he combed straight back off his forehead.

"Uh huh," I whimpered honestly. I had tried hard. My mind raced back to all the mornings I had awakened extra-early to give Wilbur milk from a bottle before I went off to school. I had not missed a morning and had never once complained, because that was the deal we had made. I kept his stall clean and Dad made me a beautiful stall sign out of wood to hang above the gate. I had lavished affection on Wilbur and spent hours and hours in the barn brushing and petting him. I could sleep on his stomach when he was lying down and I knew all his facial expressions.

Once, in deep winter, I found him after school lying outside almost frozen and unable to move. His head slumped against his almost cold body. I had been horrified and tried to get him to stand. As I pushed and pulled on him, he looked barely alive and refused to move. I ran screaming into the house, and after Dad carried Wilbur to the barn, I took warm towels and got his temperature up and stayed with him for hours until he was better. He always looked sick and scrawny, but he was all mine. I had bought him with my strawberry-picking money and, because I had spent all I'd earned for him, I didn't have many new school clothes that year. I always thought he was worth it and I spent many happy hours in the barn with him and my dad.

Eight weeks before the fair Wilbur developed an aversion to being led. No matter how I coaxed him or sternly ordered him to move, he refused to go. Standing before my father that summer day was the most difficult thing I had ever done. I was admitting failure. My parents were right, I shouldn't have tried to do something I knew nothing about. Wilbur was as ugly as my brother said he was and I would never be able to take him to the fair. All my hard work was for nothing. I began to cry harder. "I can't do it, Dad."

My father didn't say anything for a moment, he just looked at me. "Well, let's see what we can do." He swung his huge, dusty work boots off the lounge chair and headed off to the barn. I followed at his heels, suffering in silence and shame over the fact that I had been forced to ask for help.

When we arrived at the barn, Wilbur was securely tucked in a corner of his stall, chewing his cud. I ran over and threw my arms around his neck and started a new round of sobs, "Oh, Wilbur, why won't you lead!"

My dad fixed my problem that day. He hooked Wilbur to the back of the pickup truck, with his new purple halter tied to the trailer hitch, and sat me on the bumper holding the rope. He got in the front seat and hollered out the window, "Call him, sweetie, let him know you want him to come."

"Come on, Wilbur!" I shouted over the sound of the engine, "Come on!" As I urged Wilbur forward, Dad gave the truck a little gas, which tightened the rope and pulled Wilbur forward. Wilbur wasn't expecting to move and had made up his mind not to. He stiffened his legs to resist the pull, but the truck kept going and Wilbur started leaving tracks in the dirt where his hoofs were digging in. His bulging belly buckled against his back legs as the rope kept up its steady pull. Wilbur wasn't about to give up the fight that easily and figured if he refused long enough my inferior weight and leverage would win for him again. Wilbur was in for a surprise.

He twisted into a grotesque hump of black and white heaving flesh as he forced his will against the forward moving truck. As his eyes bulged out and his neck stretched out I became alarmed.

Despite his resisting, Wilbur must have realized that I had gotten a lot stronger. "Come on, Wilbur! Come on!" I shouted as, wild-eyed, he kept pulling back. I urged him to come forward. I was happy I had the truck under my seat to help me move my stubborn spoiled animal. By now, Wilbur's neck was stretched to the limit, his hooves were sliding across the ground—and then he was down! With one big thump he was on his side being dragged through the dirt with his legs kicking and a wild look in his eyes. "Daddy, he fell!" I screamed, expecting him to stop the truck at once. But it kept moving.

A voice boomed from inside the cab, "It's OK, he'll get up!" And he did. Only this time Wilbur wasn't resisting. He pulled himself up on his knees, then started jogging toward me to get closer and release the pressure of the halter

chain on his neck. I'd never seen him move so fast or grace-
fully. "Look, Daddy, he's coming! He's coming!"

We hauled Wilbur all around the pasture that day.
When we finally released him, he went quietly anywhere I
led and with only a gentle tug on his halter. It was a miracle!
His hide sported a few areas now devoid of hair, but it
would grow back.

"Daddy, how come Wilbur goes so good now?" I
asked a couple of weeks later after demonstrating my show-
manship skills. Wilbur was more behaved than any animal
I'd seen at the fair last year.

"You both just got your 'get up' back," my dad replied
with a smile.

"Our get up?" I asked.

"Yep, when something or somebody loses their get up,
sometimes they need a little help finding it again," Dad
smiled.

"I thought I wasn't supposed to ask for help. I thought
that was against the rules," I challenged him. "I failed cause
I had to get help, huh?"

"People don't fail because they ask for help, sweet-
heart, they fail because they don't ask for help."

"But, Daddy, you said…"

"I never told you I wouldn't help you," he cut me off,
"I just said you had to do the hard part, the discipline and
training part, yourself. Everybody needs to do their own
work so they can be proud of themselves, but no project is
ever done alone. I help you at the barn, don't I? And I made
you your sign."

"And you carried Wilbur in the barn when he almost
froze," I added to make him feel good.

"Yes I did. Sweetie, even the best athletes have help,
in the form of a coach or trainer. I even have a team I work

with on the job, you know." His voice was rich and pleasant. "Honey, you can't get through this life without help. Don't forget that, just know when it's time to ask for it, which you did. You waited until you had tried everything else. I'm proud of you, sweetheart, and I will always help you when you really need it."

"Thanks, Daddy," I said as I threw my arms around his waist.

Six weeks later I was standing in the show ring dressed in my crisp white jeans and shirt. Wilbur was washed and bleached and brushed until he shined. This was the breed class in which the animals were judged on conformation and marketability. The ring was round with a two-foot-high pole fence around it, bleachers on three sides and an opening on the west side facing the barns. The judge was an overweight, middle-aged man with a pot belly and a straw cowboy hat pulled down to protect his eyes from the sun. It was a hot day and my long-sleeved shirt itched and scratched under my chin as I watched the judge move each animal and owner around. He came up to each and felt the animal's flank and ran his hand down their back and side. Wilbur was acting perfect and I had my hand under his chin and was stroking his coarse chin hairs as the judge kept looking at Wilbur from the back.

Finally the judge came up and asked me in his gruff, judge's voice, "Honey, who cut this calf for you?" I was taken aback; judges never talked to you, they just judged you, and why would he ask me that?

"My dad," I replied in a tiny voice.

"Is your dad here?"

I pointed toward the opening, where my dad was standing watching with his arms crossed across his chest and a big smile for me on his face. The judge called another man over and they approached my dad as the rest of us stood in the ring in the scorching heat. My face began to flame as it seemed all eyes were trained on Wilbur and me. I didn't hear the conversation between the men and my Dad, but the judge came back and began to put each animal in its place. The ones to the farthest right would receive the blue ribbons that represented first place, then the red ribbons for second place, and the white ribbons for third and last place. You never know how many blues, reds or whites a judge will award, but you always hope for a blue. The blue also gives you the chance to go to the state fair, where only the best are allowed to compete. Wilbur led like a champ as I was directed to take the very last place on the left and was handed the only white ribbon in the class.

It seems my dad hadn't quite finished the job when he cut Wilbur to turn him from a bull into a steer. I was lucky not to be kicked out of the breed class and I felt happy because Wilbur hadn't let me down out in the ring, and we still had the showmanship competition ahead of us. I won't go into all the details of the competition, but in showmanship there is a series of classes that you must win first in order to be advanced. Wilbur and I worked so well together that we were placing first in each one. I imagine we were quite a sight, ugly, scrawny Wilbur— with his manure-stained knees that I had bleached and baby powdered to disguise—replete with his new purple show halter; and me, a little overweight, with my reddish hair pulled back into an unflattering ponytail, and freckles all over my adolescent face. I beamed as Wilbur and I were awarded the grand champion showmanship prize for my age class. The ribbon was purple and matched his halter perfectly. Wilbur had never looked so fine and I pulled my shoulders back with a newfound confidence. I had done it! I had accomplished what I set out to do, with a little help along the way, and I had finished better than I ever thought I would.

I didn't go to the fair to win ribbons; I went for the experience and the joy of working with my animal. I liked winning the purple ribbon, but I found I enjoyed the preparations even more. Wilbur had done me proud. To reward him, I gave him a little extra grain, which made his already bulging belly stick out even farther, which was just as well because as soon as he lay down in his pen, I used it for a pillow. That's where Mom and Dad found me later, snuggled in right next to Wilbur with my head on his soft white belly, as he contentedly chewed his cud.

The first "get up" lesson my dad taught me was with Wilbur, but throughout my life my dad has been my biggest influence, teaching me how to get up and get going after hardships, disappointments and defeats. I saw him do it himself, which inspired and challenged me.

Pickup #4:   Find the one who needs you.

I met my goal of going to the fair, and finished better than I thought I would because I discovered the need to help Wilbur. Most of us don't possess the motivation to do all the extras unless there is a bigger reason than merely thinking we want something. Look at your life and examine the unmet needs, and remember that when you have something external to yourself to inspire you it's easier to get going.

An example of this is owning a dog. Even when you don't want to get out of bed and go for a healthy, good-for-you walk, your pet's imploring eyes usually prevail and you take care of his needs and get up and go, which allows you to win as well.

Pickup #5:   Ask for help when you need it.

We all sometimes hit a wall in spite of our determined efforts to achieve our goals, no matter how much we want something or how big the need is. When this happens the only way to get back on track is to ask for some help. I've found that most people are glad to lend a hand when they know you are sincere. No one can motivate you unless you are ready to accept their help. As with Wilbur, a little tug can't hurt us and may help us become champions.

Pickup #6:   Do all you can with what you have.

There isn't any getting around the fact that physically, Wilbur didn't have a lot going for him. Sometimes we feel that way about ourselves. What works is to concentrate on what we do have going for us. You have inside of you the best and most efficient organ in existence, the brain and your mind. This muscle must be exercised if you want to attain your goals. Use it, expand it, fill it with good ideas and information and it will continue to push you on. You have some incredible stuff going for you; do all you can with it.

Pickup #7:   Be proud of your efforts.

Purple ribbons are nice, but usually they end up in a drawer somewhere. Pride in doing what you set out to do is displayed forever in your countenance and carriage. The best way to stay motivated is to keep moving. Be proud of all the things you do and soon the momentum will be moving you along.

So...

Find the one who needs you.

Ask for help when you need it.

Do all you can with what you have.

Be proud of your efforts.

3

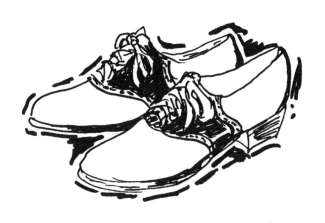

Be Open to Wonder

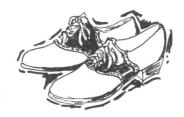

Be Open to
Wonder

We need not power or splendor,
Wide hall or lordly dome;
The good, the true, the tender,
These form the wealth of home.

—Sarah J. Hale

The room was dark, except for a tiny bit of moonlight pouring through the window and leaving a narrow beam of paleness across the foot of the beds. Kevin was in the bottom bunk and I was in the top. It was mid-December and Mom had put extra blankets on the beds to keep us warm and toasty as we slept.

"Do you think there really is a Santa?" I whispered into the darkness.

"I hope so," came Kevin's reply.

I was young enough to believe and Kevin was old enough to ask questions. I wanted desperately to believe in Santa, not so much for the presents, but for the magic. Reindeer that could fly! Imagine that.

Earlier in the day, we had gone up to our tree farm and cut down a Christmas tree. It was wet and fragrant, and Dad said we had to leave it outside for a while to dry. Mom and Kevin and I had brought out all the ornaments and we moved the furniture around so the tree would fit smack dab in front of the middle picture window in the living room. Christmas music filled the air and we bubbled with excitement and joy.

Mom had made all of the ornaments by hand, with satin balls and colorful beads. There were a lot of them and every year she added more. Sometimes she let us help her, but I didn't have the patience for it and could never seem to keep the rows of beads straight. She always complimented my childish work, and hung my half-completed ornaments somewhere on the tree.

The twinkling lights had to be unraveled and checked to see whether they were working and we had to carefully unpack the angels. This was a very special job and I had never been allowed to do it myself; this year was no exception. Mom loved her angels and didn't want them broken or chipped.

The angels continued to grow in number as the years went by. Mom would see a new one in a shop window and have to have it, or she would order them out of catalogs. She didn't do this often, though, because the angels Mom liked were porcelain and therefore expensive. Most of the angels Mom preferred were little children, seldom adults. It seemed to me a sad thing that all these children had to die to become angels, even though I knew being an angel was an important job. I believed in angels with my whole heart and every night I would pray with Mom and Kevin just so the angels would watch over me:

Matthew, Mark, Luke and John,
Bless the bed that I lie on.
Four corners to my bed
Four angels round my head.
One to watch, and one to pray
And two to bear my soul away.
Amen

Mom had found the prayer in a children's prayer book written by Dale Evans, the singing cowgirl. It was a beautiful book with lots of illustrations of country life and faith. We adopted this prayer and said it for as long as I can remember.

Mom and Dad had lots of traditions that it seemed we did forever. We prayed the same prayer before going to bed every night and before we ate dinner. We went to the Elks' family picnic every year, and Mom and Dad went hunting every fall. The normalcy and continuity kept things safe and secure for us. I don't remember how many years we did some of these things, but it seemed like we were doing them before I can remember and for as long as I recall.

Because I was already totally convinced that there were angels, I was more concerned about whether or not there was a Santa.

"Mom, is there a Santa Claus?" I knew she would tell me the truth.

"Do you believe there is one, Shawna?" I hated when she answered a question with a question, which she did a lot.

"I think so," I replied.

"If you believe there is one, then there is one," she said.

"But, is there really a Santa?" I got that whine in my voice that I used when I was confused and couldn't figure something out.

"I just told you." Mom was her calm and collected self. "Anything you believe in enough can be real for you."

I had to think about that for awhile. This thinking stuff was hard. You couldn't really know some things, you just had to think about them and figure them out in your head, which I wasn't very good at doing yet.

If what Mom said was true, and she had never lied as far as I knew, then I was the one who knew whether Santa was real. Except, I didn't know whether Santa existed, because I had never been to the North Pole. I had seen men dressed up like Santa at the mall and in different department stores, but those guys were just helping Santa out during his busy time of year. Did I need to actually see Santa to believe in him? Maybe not. I decided that Santa was real.

"I believe there's a Santa," I whispered back to Kevin.

"How come?"

"Because Mom said that if I believed in Santa, then there is a Santa—and I believe." I was strong in my conviction.

"I believe too," Kevin agreed with me, which was even more rare than going to the North Pole.

Right then, the door slowly opened and I pulled the covers up over my head to hide.

"Do I hear voices in here?" Mom's voice was also a whisper.

Kevin and I kept silent, but I moved the covers off my face to see Mom coming into the room with her hands behind her back.

"Well, you're probably asleep and don't want to see what I have." She stood very still as the covers moved in both beds and our two faces popped out to look at her.

"What, Mom?" Kevin was the first to speak.

"Just this," Mom said, and brought her hands from behind her back.

Nestled in the palm of each hand was a tiny, glowing baby angel.

The enchantment was inspiring. I rubbed my eyes to get a better look. The baby angels were no bigger than a penny. They were sitting down with their legs bent in front of them and tiny angel wings flowing off their backs. They glowed so brightly that they filled Mom's hand with light. She moved them closer to our faces and the glow filled our eyes with wonder.

Mom was beaming and cast her own kind of glow. Her surprise had worked and it was an incredible treat and a wonderful ending to a very memorable day.

"These little angels will watch over you while you sleep," she said. "I'll put one by each of your beds."

"But, Mom," I reminded her, "there's supposed to be four angels round our heads like in the prayer."

Mom took the covers and tucked them up around my chin and gave me a squeeze. "They're there," she smiled at me. "Can't you feel them?"

Suddenly I could.

There are those moments when there is nothing to say. Love filled the air with light and joy. Mom tucked us in and kissed each of us. I snuggled down into the blankets, feeling warm and contented. I believed.

Pickup #8: Believe and it will happen for you.

It doesn't matter if it's angels or Santa Claus, what we believe in becomes real for us. If you can see yourself in your mind as something you want to be, it will be more likely to happen for you because belief is a powerful motivator. Love is one of those things you can't see. We only see the demonstration of love in action. Love is something we hold inside and know, and therefore it exists because we believe it does. What do you believe?

Pickup #9:   Be open to wonder.

Little children are awed by many common and explainable things, and they are easily completely caught up in the moment. Become open to wonder and you will be astounded at how easy it is to get excited about something, how quick you are to laugh. When we forget to worry about why something is what it is, we can celebrate that it just is, which gets us looking for the things that are wondrous everywhere, wherever they come from.

Pickup #10:   Design some traditions to give stability to your life.

Every year at Christmas our family cut the tree together and we put out the angels and did the decorations. This tradition is woven into my memories so intensely that it conjures up happiness whenever something similar triggers my mind. If I get a whiff of fir trees, see an angel in a window or hear laughter, it puts me in a joyous mood. When we design our own lives and make our own traditions, we are providing ourselves and our loved ones all the opportunities they need to get motivated. We only need to move into the good places in our memories to get those same feelings no matter what the time of year. Develop some traditions to provide a place to pull from on days you're feeling down.

Pickup #11: Trust your heart to give you the answers.

Whenever I'm stumped with a problem I remember how my mother would ask me a question each time I had a question. She made me think and use my own mind to find the answers I was searching for. Too many times, I've wanted someone else to tell me what was right or what to do. I know now that only by trusting my heart and soul to provide my answers will I ever accomplish what is right for me. The answers are all inside of you; learn to trust that.

So...

Believe and it will happen for you.

Be open to wonder.

Design some traditions to give stability to your life.

Trust your heart to give you the answers.

4

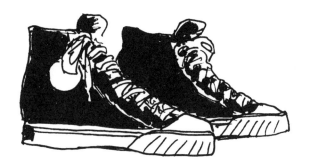

Find All the Facts

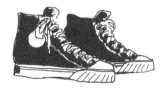

Find All the
Facts

One is not born a woman, one becomes one.
—Simone de Beauvoir

The back of my legs were sticking to the cold Formica of the bench as I sat across from Teresa Grossan during lunch. The sun was streaming through the window into the cafeteria, warming the table top where I rested my elbows while we giggled and talked. Teresa was my very best friend, which is important when you're ten and in the fifth grade. She was starting to tell me about a magazine article she had stumbled upon in her parents' room and I was giving her my full attention.

"There was this girl," she began in a whisper. I could tell it was going to be a ghost story because she had the same tone of voice we used at slumber parties and camping trips. Teresa was a farm girl and had the healthy glowing skin to prove it. She lived on a dairy farm and had rich, dark brown hair and eyes that reminded me of a baby calf.

Teresa continued, "And she was going to visit her dead mother in the graveyard one night—"

I interrupted. "Why would she go visit her mother's grave at night?"

Teresa got a huffy tone to her voice. "Probably because she worked during the day." She let out a sigh which told me my questions were unwelcome diversions.

"Now, do you want to hear the story or not?" I nodded and leaned in closer over the table.

"Well," Teresa drew a breath and exhaled, "she was kneeling at her mother's grave and it was dark and she was all alone," she paused for effect, "when this man jumped out of the bushes and grabbed her!"

My eyes were wide and she had my complete attention.

"Then he held a knife to her neck…" She was drawing the whole thing out in the way only a very young girl can— irritatingly. I touched my hand to my throat as I waited with bated breath.

"She was so scared, she threw up," she whispered with a flourish and a nervous giggle.

"She threw up on her mother's grave?" I asked in an amazed tone. I didn't know if that was a sin, but it didn't sound like the right thing to do.

"Yeah, she did," Teresa continued, "and that's not all."

I couldn't imagine anything more gross than throwing up on your mother's grave and being scared out of your wits by a guy with a knife in the middle of the night.

"Then, the guy with the knife…" Teresa gave another dramatic pause, "he put his in hers!" She looked at me very knowingly.

I was confused. "His what?" I asked.

"His 'thing,'" she giggled.

I still didn't get it. I had never seen a man's "thing," and this wasn't making any sense to me at all. More importantly, I was becoming quite shocked by this information.

"Where did he put his thing?" I fiercely whispered.

"I told you, he put his thing in her thing," she said.

My face was a picture of confusion and revulsion. "We don't have a 'thing,'" I shot back, knowing she was wrong.

"I know, stupid," she said in a worldly voice. "But we have a place."

"You mean where we pee?" My lips curled like I'd just eaten a slug and my stomach felt like it.

"The other place." She rolled her eyes.

Wow. My head was reeling and I was more horrified than I had ever been before. There was another place? And "his thing" could fit in it. I shuddered. I didn't want to appear naive, but this information was so far beyond anything I had even considered that I was dumbfounded and speechless.

"And she just kept throwing up and everything!" Teresa added, which I guessed ended the story she said she had read in a magazine.

"That's horrible. Why would he do that?" I demanded. Visions of graveyards, knives and vomit floated in fast procession through my confused and frightened brain.

Teresa got that knowing tone in her voice again, "Because that's how people have babies, stupid!"

She had gone over the line. "No they don't!" I screeched. Babies were about good things. There was no way those vile ideas could have anything to do with babies.

"Yes sir!" Teresa seemed quite convinced that her horrid story was true, and like a lot of girls in the fifth grade, she wanted to prove how much she knew about life. "My mom says she and Dad do it all the time and that Dad is heavy." She giggled again and took a sip from her milk carton.

My mind was reeling and I felt like I would vomit as I assembled this information in my ten-year-old head. Suddenly, Teresa's father, whom I had barely acknowledged in the past, became a sinister character I envisioned jumping from bushes and smashing poor Mrs. Grossan to death. "Well," I said through clenched teeth, "my mom and dad would never do anything like that."

"I bet they do," she sneered. " My mom says all married people do."

I didn't know what married people did, I had never cared, but I knew without a shadow of a doubt that my mom and dad would never do anything like that. "No they don't!" I almost screamed, trying to cling to something, anything. "That's why I'm adopted!"

Finally a saving thought. That was it! I was right after all. If babies came from doing something so awful, then it was only natural that my decent parents had adopted us. I hung on to that thought all afternoon as the day sped by and I sat through class like a zombie. When I got off the bus, which stopped a quarter of a mile from my house, I ran all the way home.

I was out of breath and visibly upset as I burst into the kitchen, where my mother and dad were sitting enjoying the afternoon sun.

"Mom! I need to talk to you—now!" I was breathing hard and had a wild look in my eye. I had to get to the bottom of this right away.

"What's wrong, honey?" Mom was alert to my mood.

"I can't tell you here!" I glanced at Dad, the man—the enemy—out of the corner of my eye. "Please come to the bathroom!" I turned on my heel and ran down the hall to the bathroom door. Mom came hurrying down the hall behind me and as she came through the door I slammed it behind her and threw myself against it, panting. Mom went over to the toilet, put the lid down and sat.

"What's the matter, honey?" she asked quietly.

Now that I had her there, what was I supposed to say? What if she didn't know that people did this…this…thing? How do I tell her this awful stuff? The tears welled up behind my eyes as I came forward to face my mom.

"Mom, Teresa told me something at lunch today." My voice didn't sound like my own.

"What was it, honey?" Mom encouraged me.

The words rushed out of my mouth like greyhounds released for a race. "Teresa told me that boys put their things in girls' things and that this man did that to a girl on her mother's grave and she threw up and that's how babies are born and that every married couple does it and that her parents do it and I said that mine would never do that and that's why I'm adopted." Finally I took a breath.

The tears began as I gazed at my mother, hoping that she would take away this knowledge, that she would tell me Teresa was wrong and I was right and that the world could go back to the way it had been before lunch.

"You don't do that, do you, Mom?" I implored her with my whole body. "Tell me you and Daddy don't do that, Mom." I sank to my knees and placed my head on her lap and let the tears flow more freely. Mom stroked my hair and tried to comfort me while she hid her smile.

My mother is a very smart woman. She waited until she was forty to adopt me; or I should say she didn't have the opportunity to adopt me until she was forty. Some people think that's too old to become a mother, that you need to be younger to have the energy, but my mom had enough wisdom to cover all the bases in the very best way.

"You don't do that, do you, Mom?" I asked again though tear-filled eyes. The fact that she hadn't denied it immediately was worrisome. Mom took my face between her wonderful warm hands and looked deep into my eyes. Then, without saying a word, she nodded.

The truth was staring at me, and in my mother's eyes it wasn't quite as hard to take, but I was stricken with despair anyway and began to cry harder.

"Why, Mom?" I sobbed. "Why would you do such a terrible thing?"

"Shawna." My mother said my name in a soft and loving way. I didn't look up, my sobs becoming more pronounced as I realized how stupid I was.

"Shawna, look at me." She took my face in her hands again and wiped away my tears. "I'm going to ask you something and I want you to answer me."

I gazed at her, then averted my eyes. I was being betrayed by someone I thought I knew.

"Shawna, have I ever lied to you?" Mom asked me in a firmer tone. I didn't reply.

"Shawna, I'm asking you a question and I want you to answer it." Her voice got stronger and she gently squeezed my face. "Have I ever lied to you?"

I glumly shook my head no; she had never lied to me.

"Well I'm going to tell you the truth right now and even if you don't believe it now, I'm not lying and I never will lie to you, all right?" She gave me a little smile.

This was a very serious moment and I was filled with so many emotions and confusions. I grabbed Mom as if she were my lifeline.

"What Teresa told you about was a bad thing. Someone being grabbed at her mother's grave shouldn't happen to anyone. That is really terrible. When married couples are together it isn't a bad thing, it's a beautiful thing." She was talking to me as I began to shake my head no.

"I will never do that! Never, never, never!" I sobbed. "If married people do that, then I am never getting married, ever!"

"Shawna, when you meet the right person and fall in love you will want to do that," Mom told me.

"No I won't!" I set my chin. "I will never want to do that, ever!"

Mom was firm and paused until I calmed down a little. "I promise you, Shawna, and I have never broken a promise have I?" She waited. "Have I?"

"No," came a little voice from me.

"Well I promise you that when you meet the right person, you will want to do this; and more importantly, you will like it very much." She smiled again.

"No I won't—" I started to say again, but she interrupted me.

"Trust me in this, honey; I promise you." I sniffed and let her scoop me up in her arms. This was a warm and wonderful place. My mother was soft and gentle and was a haven whenever I was down. I let her cuddle me and soothe me as I had myself a very good cry.

Things changed between us after that day. I look back on it now and realize that was when I grew past childhood and started the journey into adolescence. Mom became my ally and my confidant and I knew I could ask her anything, having asked her about the terrible story. I was firm in my belief that I would never do the thing married people did and that I wouldn't marry, but I became curious about things after that. For several years, each time I saw couples together I would question Mom.

"They don't do it, do they, Mom?" I would inquire when the man was a huge, towering guy and his wife was five foot two.

"I'm sure they do," Mom would always reply.

"How?" I'd ask.

She was always evasive and mysterious. "Oh, there's ways."

One day when we were alone in the house, I questioned her. "Mom, what do boys' 'things' look like?"

Mom seemed surprised but gave me a smile. She didn't answer right away, probably because she was lost for words. How do you describe it?

"Have you ever seen George's?" Mom asked me. George was our overweight and elderly Black Labrador.

My eyes got wide and my lip rolled up in disgust. "It's pink and pointy and comes out of his hairy part?" I asked in bafflement. I never considered that the thing would resemble a dog's thing, especially old decrepit George's.

"Forget I said that," Mom quickly countered. "Let me think about it, OK, honey?"

I nodded agreement and went out to find George for another look.

Several weeks later when we were alone again, Mom took me aside,

"Do you still want to see what a man's 'thing' looks like?" she asked me.

I pondered for a moment. I hadn't thought about it since the dog comparison had happened. As a matter of fact, I tried never to think about it. Yuck! But my curiosity was aroused and other girls my age knew what it looked like. I'd been living in a house with my dad and brother my whole life and I had never seen one, ever. So I nodded to Mom.

"Come on then." She started down the hall to her and Dad's room. When we got to the door, she stopped just outside, where we had some built-in shelves above built-in drawers. She pulled out the bottom drawer and, using it as a step, reached up to the top shelf and pulled out a magazine. She left the drawer out and we went into her room. We crawled onto the bed on our stomachs, side by side, and Mom opened the magazine. Inside were pictures of naked men displaying their "things."

Several years had passed since I had heard the story from Teresa and by now I was a preteen and quite a bit more mature. Mom and I had developed quite a wonderful relationship and the day we pored over a skin magazine together became a good memory in my mind. My fifty-something mother had used a lot of guts and courage to buy that magazine in our small town and even more to handle my questions.

Mom was given the gift of mothering, and also the pain of not being able to give birth to a child. Instead, she gave birth to my imagination and spirit. She was not only a kind and thoughtful mother, but a friend, someone who loved me enough to always tell the truth, even when it wasn't easy or pretty. Her promise to me about finding someone to love and enjoying the sexual experience was a huge gift. As usual, her promise was good.

Pickup #12: Find someone who will tell you the truth.

My mother never lied to me, so when she promised that someday I would understand and that I would change my mind it gave me hope. We all need to find people in our lives who aren't afraid to tell us the truth and help us find the courage to move past our present circumstances. We also must be willing to believe those who do tell us the truth even when it's not what we want to hear. Motivation comes from involving your mind and heart; you must be open-hearted to grow.

Pickup #13: Be open to learning all things even when they appear unpleasant at first.

I was determined that I would never marry because I learned about sex in a disgusting way. How many times have we formed an opinion without really knowing all the facts? Learning to move past your prejudices and being open to learn more about something places you in a good position to make decisions and to get going with your life.

Pickup #14: Recognize that you are not stupid if you don't know something.

Young girls want to think they are sophisticated and worldly so they may at times put someone else down to appear superior. Young girls, of course, are not the only ones who do this. When we realize that not knowing something doesn't make us stupid, it just gives us an opportunity to learn something, we let go of the fear that we will do or say the wrong thing. Keep asking questions and you will learn things you don't know, then you will begin to outshine those doing all the talking.

Pickup #15: Have a good cry when you're disappointed.

Whenever it rained (and it rains a lot in Oregon), my mother would say it was as though God had reached down and wiped off the face of the earth. "A fresh start," my mother would say when I was having a darn good cry. Sometimes we need to wash away the pain and confusion. The best way I've found is a good cry, which makes me feel as though God has come down and wiped off my face. Then I can make a fresh start and I can keep going.

So...

Find someone who will tell you the truth.

Be open to learning all things even when they appear unpleasant at first.

Recognize that you are not stupid if you don't know something.

Have a good cry when you're disappointed.

5

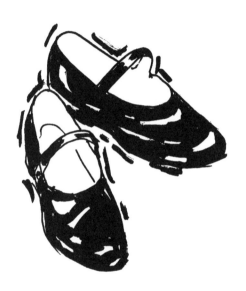

Do the Right Thing

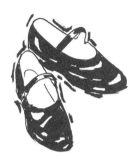

Do the Right Thing

Truth never hurts the teller.

—Robert Browning

We lived in a house that Dad had built before he and Mom knew that they would adopt us kids, so it was small and cozy. Two bedrooms and four of us. Mom always said that the carpet and drapes were temporary—for sixteen years they were temporary.

I'll never forget when Mom finally convinced Dad to spring for some new furniture. She was so excited, she was like a little kid and spent hours analyzing and selecting until she decided on a French Provincial set, with one coffee table and two end tables, a very big deal.

Our living room was long and wide. The house faced southwest and had huge, floor-to-ceiling picture windows along the front side, which revealed an unbelievable view of the valley our house sat above. Because the sun set in the west, these windows had drapes that closed to form a full wall of curtains, which prevented the sun from streaming in and ruining Mom's precious furniture in the afternoons. On most days Mom only opened the drapes to uncover the center bank of windows and I often wondered why they bothered to have all those windows when they almost always kept the drapes shut.

I opened the drapes as wide as they would go whenever I got the chance, and always when I was in the house alone. At night, if I left every light on in the living room and opened the drapes as wide as I could, the windows formed a mirror backdrop that reflected my fledgling teenage body as I discovered my love of dance and performance.

I suspect that more teenage girls would have better self-esteem and confidence if they could spend uninter-rupted time moving and playing in front of a wall of window mirrors on late Friday and Saturday nights and at other times when there isn't anyone to tell them to turn the music down or turn off some of the lights. You shouldn't have to worry about the electric bill when you're learning how to be something other than someone's daughter.

When Mom bought the new furniture, Kevin and I were preteens and still into fighting and competition. We've never outgrown this, by the way. Anyway, when the new furniture came, Mom sat Kevin and me down and gave us a "talking to." Some would call it a lecture, but at our house it was a "talking to." During a talking to, Mom and Dad were the only ones allowed to do the talking. Kevin and I were the talkees.

We got talked to about strangers, safety, and proper table manners, as well as anything else my parents deemed important. After many years of getting talked to, we ceased to listen much. Most of the subjects were of no interest to us. What did they think, that we had just fallen off a turnip truck or something? We knew better than to go with someone we didn't know, we knew guns weren't toys, and we knew Mom's new furniture was important and not to whack it with the vacuum cleaner.

One day Kevin and I were in the kitchen arguing about something when Mom came storming in, red in the face and breathing hard. The look in her eyes was murderous and her fists were clenched in a threatening way. Kevin and I both shrank back into the shelter of the kitchen chairs as Mom came unglued.

"All right, which one of you wrote on my new furniture!" Mom shot a fiery glance at me and then at Kevin. Her body was heaving and she was having trouble controlling herself.

Kevin and I weren't stupid. We saw her condition, we feared for our lives, we lied.

"Not me!" Kevin shouted, looking innocent and sweet, and beating me to the punch.

"Not me neither!" I added as Mom's face got redder and I tried to disappear into the cushion of the kitchen seat.

Mom glared from one to the other of us and didn't say a word. The minutes seemed suspended in time and I could hear her heart pounding—or was it my heart? I had never seen Mom so mad, and I didn't know where to turn. I knew we were in trouble and I didn't know what to do. I looked over at Kevin, who wouldn't meet my eyes, and waited.

My mother is a very smart cookie; she proved it to me dozens of times. After the strong denial from both of us, she stopped in her tracks and realized that we weren't going to admit to anything that would cause us bodily harm. She drew in a long, hard breath and let it out slowly between her teeth as she unclenched her fists.

"All right," she said in a much calmer tone of voice.

"I know one of you wrote on the new furniture, and I'm very unhappy about it, but..." she paused and looked pointedly at each of us, "I will not have my children lying to me." She stated her decision as a matter of fact. "So, this is what I am going to do."

It was obvious from her tempered approach that the Mom we knew and loved was coming back. I could see the wheels working in her brain. My mom was so consistent, so loving, and I was so glad to see that the furniture incident hadn't completely taken away her senses.

"Whichever one of you did this, I want you to tell me. I won't punish you for it, but it's very important that I know." She waited.

I breathed a sigh of relief. I knew I hadn't done it, which put me off the hook, and it looked as though Kevin wouldn't be in too much trouble.

She wasn't finished with us yet. "I can forgive you for making a mistake on the furniture." She had an edge to her voice I hadn't heard before. "But if you lie to me..." She paused again for effect (my mother should have been a dramatic actress), "you will be punished." The threat was out. She had set the rules and I knew she meant business.

"It wasn't me," Kevin insisted, and looked down at his eggs.

I was stunned. I was mortified, horrified. I couldn't believe my ears as Mom smiled at Kevin and turned her cold, steely eyes on me.

"It wasn't me neither!" I exclaimed, too loud and too high. I sounded like I was lying, even to myself.

Mom straightened up and set her chin. She could not conceal her displeasure.

"All right then," she sighed. "Let's just go look at the furniture."

OK, I thought, this will prove without a shadow of a doubt that I'm innocent. I had not written on the furniture, and had no idea how or where the infraction had occurred, so I sprang willingly out of the chair I was glued to and followed her into the living room. The drapes were shut.

Mom marched us over to one of the end tables and stood with her legs apart and her hands folded in front of her chest. She glanced down and there, embedded in the soft wood of the new French Provincial end table, was a small, tiny word that looked as if it had been written on a piece of paper so thin that the pen had pushed through it, leaving a defacing mark on the gleaming surface of Mom's pride and joy. Whoever had done the writing had no doubt realized that the pen had left a mark because there was only the one word and nothing more.

I looked down at the mark, expecting to be vindicated, expecting to have proof without a shadow of a doubt that it was Kevin who was lying, and that I deserved Mom's forgiveness and her love. What I saw made my heart sink. There, embedded in the wood on Mom's new end table, was one undeniable word, "Shawna."

"Well?" my mom looked at the two of us.

"Mom, I didn't write on this, I swear." I implored her to believe me.

"Me neither," Kevin said.

I couldn't believe this was happening.

My mom was clearly disappointed in both of us and her eyes took on a hurt and defeated look.

"I will forgive whoever did this if you will just not lie to me." She was giving us another chance to confess without fear.

My whole body wanted to confess just to receive Mom's forgiveness, to have her take me in her arms and

love me, but I couldn't. A big tear found its way out of the
corner of my eye and slid down my cheek. I wanted Mom's
love but not with a lie. I remained silent and so did Kevin.
She left the room and went into her bedroom and shut the
door, leaving us alone together in front of the end table.

"Why didn't you tell her you did this?" I spat out at
Kevin the minute I heard Mom's door shut.

"Because I didn't do it, stupid," Kevin said. He had
that "I told you so" tone that I hated. "It's your name, isn't
it?" He knew there wasn't anything I could say.

Kevin and I had completely different philosophies
when it came to our parents. I was forever seeking love and
attention; I craved it, demanded it and couldn't get enough.
My biggest fear growing up was that I would make a huge
mistake and they would give me back.

Kevin figured that since his biological mother hadn't
wanted him, probably nobody else did either, and he was
setting out to prove himself right. Kevin continually gave
Mom and Dad a hard time; he always bucked their authority
and tested their temper. I would watch in horror as he said
and did things that certainly should have gotten him sent
back to wherever he came from. But our parents loved us
through whatever came their way. They never treated us as
adopted; we were theirs, good or bad. Kevin needed their
love proved constantly and so he acted out; I needed their
love proved constantly and acted as perfect as I could. What
neither of us realized is that we didn't need to act any which
way to be totally loved, we just were.

The lie was never confessed as far as I know. We got
older, the furniture acquired other battle scars from guests
and general use. No one ever wrote on it again, but my
name is still embedded on one end table. I never lied to my
parents and I know Kevin did. The differences between us

grew from that day on and I learned that sometimes even when you're right it's not enough to fix a situation, and no matter how hard you work at doing the best thing it's sometimes not enough.

I also learned that it doesn't really matter whether someone believes you or not as long as you know you've done the right thing. The reverse is certainly true as well: even if you get away with a lie you know the truth in your heart. I would like to believe that living with a lie is worse than getting away with telling it.

Whether Mom believed me or not is no longer important, I know I was innocent and I know that not confessing just to win approval or love was the right thing to do. I can live with that.

Pickup #16: Do the right thing no matter what the circumstances.

It's always tempting to do or say what other people want to hear because then you know they will like you and be happy with you and there won't be any waves. The challenge in this is that you have to live with knowing that you weren't honest with yourself or them. Doing the right thing isn't always the easy thing, but it's the only way to keep getting up. If you allow the wrong things to happen too often soon you are stuck in a self-created mire. Do the right thing and you will gain the power to proceed.

Pickup #17: Always talk "with" people.

When someone is "talked to" they usually cease to listen. The wrong kind of lecture is the surest way to shut another person's mind. Engage the people you are having conversations with, including children and peers. Ask questions, compliment and encourage, and the energy that comes back to you will give you an incredible boost. Want to get some energy? Spend some on someone else and it doubles!

Pickup #18: Open the drapes and let the sun in!

My mother's furniture seemed more important to her than allowing the sun to fill the room. What priority do you have that is preventing you from letting joy into your life? My husband and I have built a new log home with huge picture windows and not a drape in the place, so the sun and rain can pound on the windows and fill us with the gumption it takes to get going. Sometimes you must open yourself up to let the sun come in.

Pickup #19: Forgive and move on.

Even though neither my brother nor I told Mom that we had made a mistake, I learned that I would have been forgiven. The best lesson in getting over something is knowing that you can be forgiven and move past whatever mistake you've made. Not admitting to a lie or mistake can make you sick and sluggish, but taking responsibility and facing the consequences can add another layer of pride and confidence around you that will help you next time you err. Soon the mistakes will diminish in magnitude, and be mere stumbles along life's road.

So...

Do the right thing no matter what the circum-
stances.

Always talk "with" people.

Open the drapes and let the sun in!

Forgive and move on.

6

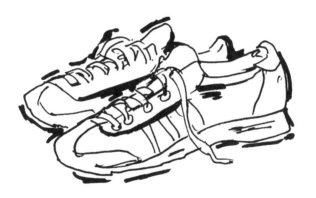

Stand Your Ground

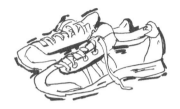

Stand Your Ground

I hear and I forget. I see and I remember. I do and I understand.

—Chinese proverb

"Get out—now!" My dad's voice sounded like a clap of thunder inside the stillness of the pickup cab. I set my teeth, squared my shoulders and gripped the wheel.

"No."

Complete silence followed. To say no to my dad was quite a feat and I didn't know what to expect next. There we were in the middle of nowhere and I was disobeying my father for the first time. Pretty heady stuff for a fourteen-year-old girl. The air was filled with tension. I think we were both surprised by my defiance.

That morning I had been just a normal teenager, thinking about unimportant stuff like boys, school, dance, boys, those really terrific shoes Mom wouldn't let me get, and boys. I'm not certain when I became so boy crazy, but I think it started sometime the previous summer when we went to the annual Elks picnic and this really cute guy started paying attention to me. It was particularly flattering because he was so worldly and mature. He could drive already and even had his own truck! He got me thinking about stuff that had never even crossed my mind before, like how I acted and sounded and what it might be like to be kissed.

After that summer, I started to think about boys a lot. I also concluded that my social situation was incredibly bleak. I lived out in the middle of the country with my parents and my stone-headed brother, who was two years older and was allowed to do almost everything. I, on the other hand, practically had to ask to go to the bathroom! Two years older and he could drive around with Dad and stay after school. Life was so unfair!

Sometime during this period, I decided I would begin a little early preparing for the wonderful time I would have when I could drive my own car and have a social life. So I started in on my dad, "Dad, remember how you let Kevin drive when no one was around?"

"Yep." My dad was preoccupied.

"When did you start letting him do that do you think?" I asked him in my sweetest voice.

"Honey, I don't remember," he said. "Why?"

OK, now we were getting somewhere.

"Well, I was thinking that since you did such a good job teaching Kevin, maybe you might teach me?" Flattery usually worked. Even though I was only fourteen, I had my dad pretty much figured out.

"Well…"

He was on the edge, I could tell.

"Daddy, don't you believe in me?" I was going in for the kill.

"Of course I believe in you, honey, but you are only fourteen."

Weak argument; he was slipping fast.

"You said yourself I was mature for my age. Didn't you mean it?" My pleading look and slight quiver in the lip were calculated to seal the deal.

"Well, OK, I'll let you drive next time we go up for wood."

Triumph filled my body but I tilted my head down and acted shy, "Thank you, Daddy." I was on the road to freedom!

I have always wondered whether my dad put off going to get wood just to make me stew about it for two weeks. Finally, the day arrived that we were going up to the property for wood. Just me and Dad. An hour to get there and an hour to get back. I could hardly contain my excitement. The only negative aspect of the experience was the vehicle. Whenever my dad went to get wood, he took the old blue truck. This truck was a nightmare to ride in, and now as I began to view it as an inexperienced driver, I started to have second thoughts.

First of all, it was a stick shift, and this stick came out of the floor panel at a slightly different angle than the manufacturer intended, which caused it to shoot away from the steering wheel farther than my arm could reach. The steering wheel itself was something to behold. It was an extra large version, the kind you used to see in all the older trucks. I swear it had never seen a wash rag during its entire existence and it was caked with grime and dried coffee and who knows what else.

The whole inside of the cab was like that and had a musty smell to it. The smell came from a variety of sources, like half-eaten lunches left too long behind the seat, and coffee, pop and liquor spilled on the floor. There was also the odor of gun oil mingled with wet dog smell in the seat.

The worst thing of all was the seat. My dad is a carpenter and used this truck for work. He must have jumped in a lot of times without taking off his tool belt, because the seat looked like a varmint had chewed on it just on the driver's side. There were holes and gashes and foam coming out all over. My backside could probably fit into one of the holes, they were so big. The only other features I've failed to describe were the mold on the ceiling and the clutter on the dash. This truck was a beauty all right, and in this monstrosity I was going to have my first driving lesson. I could hardly wait!

All the way up to the property I pestered Dad. He couldn't seem to find just the right place to pull over, or there were too many people on the road. When we reached our destination, I hadn't even sat behind the wheel. I was a very unhappy girl. So I refused to talk to him the whole time we loaded wood. Nothing gets at my dad worse than not talking to him.

Most people would be intimidated by my dad. He is really big and broad. He has big strong arms and can do practically anything. He hunts and fishes and chops wood. He always makes me feel very protected and loved. He tried everything that day to make me laugh. He made funny faces, he turned the radio up and danced around. I almost gave in to him because he was trying so hard, but this issue was too important to give in. I needed to drive to have any kind of life. I had to drive or I would be forever stuck in the country and turn into an old maid. I wasn't even doing it just for me. I knew that I couldn't burden my folks with driving me everywhere. I was really being selfless in this pursuit. Really!

On the way back, I tried a new tactic: silence, punctuated with long, audible sighs. As we neared the section of road I thought would be perfect for my first lesson, I let out

▬ ▪ ▬ ▪ ▬ ▪ ▬ ▪ ▬ ▪ ▬ ▪ ▬ ▪ ▬ ▪ ▬ ▪ ▬ ▪ ▬ ▪ ▬

a big sigh that said, I guess you don't really love me. By now I figured my dad would be ready for my last tactic. "You said you would teach me to drive next time we went for wood—you promised!" (Just a faint catch in the throat.) "Aren't you gonna?" I reached over and touched his arm.

"OK, you win! But if you see anyone on the road I want you to stop this truck!"

"But Dad—" I began.

"Now I mean it! This is very dangerous and you have to promise me if you see anyone, anyone at all, you will stop this truck immediately! Promise me, or you don't drive!"

He seemed pretty set so I murmured a faint "OK." I remember the feelings of anticipation and excitement that mingled with terror and fear as I traded places with him. Could I drive this monster? What if I killed us? I climbed into the driver's side. I had to sit all the way on the front of the seat so my feet could reach the pedals—and so I wouldn't fall into a hole in the seat.

"OK, put in the clutch and press the brake at the same time," he instructed.

Whoa, this was hard! I had to grab that grimy steering wheel in a bear hug to position myself to push down on the pedals.

"Let it out slow now."

Pop! The truck bucked like a horse and the engine went out. I glanced over at my dad.

"I said slow!" he barked. "Try it again."

I must admit that first lurch forward scared me a tiny bit, but no harm done. I started the process over. This time I let the clutch out much slower, but I didn't let my other foot off the brake. No gas, no go. Pop! Dead again. This was much harder than I envisioned.

"Honey, are you sure you want to do this?" my dad asked in a quieter voice.

That was all it took to set my mind and will. I wasn't going to let this truck beat me. This old smelly, holey-seated relic. This was my life we were talking about here. If I gave up now, Dad might never let me have another chance.

"I can do it, Daddy, I know I can." I gave him a winning smile and clutched the steering wheel harder.

"OK, baby, let's do it again."

He did believe in me!

"Now remember," he warned, "if you see anyone, anyone at all, coming on this road you stop right away, OK?"

"I promise," I assured him and finally I got the darn thing rolling. After the clutch was let out and I was pushing the gas, it wasn't that tough, really. The steering took some getting used to, but I kept the truck pretty much on my side of the road.

Then it happened. I was concentrating on the road so hard, and staying on my side, that the other car seemed to come from nowhere toward me. Dad didn't even see it, but I did, and I remembered my promise right away. I suppose we should have practiced stopping before I was called on to do it. I didn't know you were supposed to put in that nasty old clutch. I just slammed on the brakes. Of course, I knew I was stopping, so my arms took most of the jolt. Dad, however, was watching me, so when the truck stopped, he didn't.

Whatever clutter had been on the dash was now on either Dad, me or the floor. I think he broke a coffee mug with his arm or an elbow. As red as he got in the face, I'm surprised he didn't have a heart attack.

"Get out—now!" he thundered, which brings us to the moment of defiance: that small, iron-willed "No," which came out of my mouth almost of its own accord. As I sat there breathing hard, waiting for what my dad might do, I decided a good offense was better than a weak defense.

"You told me to stop. You said no matter what, if I saw somebody, to stop immediately. You told me to and I did it. I was only doing what you told me to do."

I didn't look at him; I just stared straight ahead hoping that the logic I was using would work. Out of the corner of my eye I saw him reach down to the floor. My body tensed. He brought up his old hard hat from work and placed it on his head.

"Start it up," he said between clenched teeth.

Inwardly I smiled. I could do this, I really could.

Pickup #20: Don't give up until you get what you want.

People don't know what you want or how bad you want it unless you tell them. If you want something as bad as I wanted to learn to drive you will learn to use all the tactics you can think of and ones you aren't even aware of. Using silence, nagging, or appealing to someone's sense of right or wrong are all tactics we can use to let someone know we mean business. There are many ways to do something; try them all until you get what you want.

Pickup #21: Try things even when you're scared of them.

That truck was a monster and a means to an end. I was terrified to drive it but my desire for freedom was greater than the fear of getting behind that wheel. Instead of deciding immediately that you will or won't try something, figure out what you will gain from the experience. That way the fear you feel can fuel your desire instead of dampen it.

Pickup #22:   Learning to stop is as important as learning to go.

In my zeal to get behind the wheel, I never practiced stopping and that got me in trouble. When I was learning to ski, the instructor spent considerable time teaching us how to stop. To pick up your get up is great, but sometimes you must stop as well, so you can get up and go again.

So...

Don't give up until you get what you want.

Try things even when you're scared of them.

Learning to stop is as important as learning to go.

7

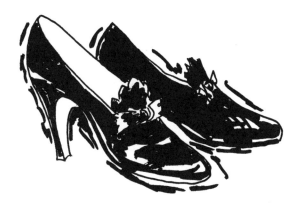

Take Risks

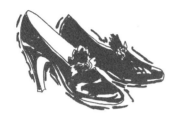

Take Risks

To live is like to love—all reason is against it, and all healthy instinct is for it.

—Samuel Butler

Judging from my dad's face, there was more wrong with the road show equipment truck than its looks. He tried to remain calm and unconcerned as more and more bags and equipment were loaded into the decrepit old vehicle.

"Where do you keep the spare tire on this thing?" Dad attempted some conversation with one of the musicians.

"Gee," came a voice from the recesses of the back, "I don't even know if we have a spare tire."

My dad started to pace as we watched my own bags get loaded in. I was too consumed with excitement to pay Dad much mind. I was finally beginning my life. It didn't matter to me that it was starting out in a rusted and badly-in-need-of-paint former U-haul truck. I just knew that I was going somewhere, and anywhere seemed better than nowhere.

"Why don't you think about going to school and working for awhile?" my mom tentatively asked me as I signed up for the last of my required high school classes at the local community college.

"Since I loathed high school, I guess it would seem logical to you if I decided to sign up for four more years, huh Mom?" I was being cheeky, which she hated.

"Well, you could get a job and work for a while and get a nice little apartment, wouldn't you like that?" She was trying to keep me in town.

"Mom," I changed my tone to help her understand just how important this decision was to me, "I only have this one life and I intend to live it with every shred of gusto I've got." My voice took on passion and excitement. "I want to go places and see things and meet other types of people." Then, because I knew my leaving was hurting her, I got sorta quiet. "I can't live here until I know what's out there."

Looking like she might cry, my mother left the room. I sat for a minute thinking about what I had just said. I had no idea what the future held in store for me, but I did know without a shadow of a doubt that, if I didn't pick up and get going now, I might never live the way I wanted to. I had to risk it.

My life at home had turned into one big question. "What are you going to do now?" I had been dancing for years, taking every class offered and several that weren't. I had given up years of fun activities in order to be a dancer; how was I going to justify all the sacrifices? Could I just leave it behind and get a teaching certificate? Lots of dancers did. Maybe I should move to L.A., attempt to land a job performing somewhere, and join the millions of aspiring actors, dancers and who knows who else living down there.

The question I kept asking myself was, "Is dancing all there is?" I didn't really like my options. I wanted to dance, act, sing, shout, and be one hundred percent alive. But how? Going on the road seemed like the only way I could be a performer, travel and see the world, keep my clothes on, and discover what and who I was.

The choices I had locally didn't excite me. On the fringes of the only large city in Oregon, if you can call Portland large, there aren't a lot of legitimate job openings for a young, impressionable dancer with performance talent, drive, and no common sense, who doesn't want to strip for a living.

I begged my dance instructor, who had witnessed the sacrifices I had made to dance, to help me find a job performing. "What would you do?" I asked her.

Gail sighed. "I would go," she said. My wonderful Miss Gail, the instructor who gave me my beat, who believed in me, who had the patience and skill to help a little nobody from Helvetia to dream.

"How?" I demanded, before pouring out my tale of woe. There wasn't any money; Dad had been sick and Mom was pulling the weight with the finances. My parents didn't want me to leave home, my boyfriend didn't want me to leave home. I didn't know a soul anywhere outside of Oregon. I even had a dog I didn't know what to do with. Hopelessness and defeat began to batter my usually unconquerable spirit.

"Maybe I'm not good enough." I played a card that would either help me or hinder me.

"You are," Gail said. "Let me make some calls."

The audition Gail set up was with an old dancing buddy of hers who, along with her gentlemen friend, had a traveling show band. They needed a singer, dancer and entertainer to back up the lead guy, who was her boyfriend. I got the job.

The first thing I noticed was that I was so far over my head it was like walking in rubber boots through cow manure. Think stinky and difficult. I was Little Miss Purity thrust smack dab into the middle of musician decadence.

The band members were road warriors from way back. Joey, from New York, talked with a heavy Brooklyn accent, had pock-marked skin and Afro-curled hair. Eddie from Miami, tall, dark and exotic, played the piano and used his looks to get his way with both men and women. Duane, the drummer, was quiet and shy, with a groove you could move to. I don't remember the bass player, but I do remember the light and sound man, Mark, who was Polish, performed mime, and had signed on to see the world, just like me. Another girl sang and danced, and together she and I were the backdrop for the lead man.

Thus began my first experience with raw human nature wrapped in egos the size of our run-down truck. The band members didn't so much work together as we worked at the same time—each for his or her own agenda. We were each there for our own reasons, and making the show successful wasn't one of them. Even as young as I was, I knew we had some serious communication problems and no common goal. One thing I knew for certain: I wasn't in Oregon anymore.

We worked in dives and good places (the kind I always knew existed), making money one week and owing them my paycheck the next, for gas to get us to the next gig. I didn't know how we got booked or what was expected of me, and I trusted everyone. My mistake.

This initial experience left me somewhat disillusioned with show biz. I loved the travel, the people and the performing. I didn't much like the band guys or the other girl in the show, and I learned definitely not to trust the leader of the band.

Show bands are a strange and interesting phenomenon. They fill in the void between the big, flashy stage shows and ordinary lounge bands. Our show had wild costumes, great lighting effects and choreographed numbers. We went to entertain instead of just play music.

I called home often to tell about the exotic places I was seeing, and the strange sights and accents, but I didn't talk much about the show and Mom got wise to me.

We were up in Anchorage, Alaska, at the Holiday Inn, where I would be spending Christmas. I spent the next five Christmases away from home, but this was the first, and every time I called my parents it was painful.

On the twentieth of December, or so, I was busily preparing for a show when the front desk called to say that a package had been delivered and would I please come down and get it.

"I can't come down now," I lamented into the phone. "My hair's in rollers and I'm already late. Can't someone bring it up?"

This, for some reason, was impossible and they insisted I come down right away to get my unusual package. They wouldn't tell me where it was from, though I could guess, and they were insistent that I hurry down before the show and get it. I was exasperated but threw something on and headed down the stairs with curlers still in my hair.

Mom was standing at the front desk holding a Christmas tree she had obviously hauled all the way from Oregon. I squealed with delight. I couldn't believe what a wonderful surprise this was, but I was late, so I grabbed her bags and herded her up the stairs.

Mom only stayed for three days and she went home in time to spend Christmas with Dad and Kevin, but it sure made my holiday to have her visit me. She watched a lot while she was there and knew I wasn't doing what I really wanted, but what could she do to help me? Not much.

Six months of constant travel and performance would change anyone. I had gone on the road as a naive, young, country girl from Oregon. I had soft hair and makeup, a conservative manner and a shy but intense personality. I wanted to make sure those folks back home knew I had grown up, that I was living my dream. I got a wild full-curl perm, loaded on the makeup and put a fake tattoo on my neck. When Dad picked me up I had on skintight, bright red disco pants (this was the late seventies) and a wild polyester shirt unbuttoned to my bra. Dad took one look and said, "Please get back on the plane and come off as my daughter this time."

I roared with laughter. "Daddy, what's the matter?" My goal had been to shock him. "Don't you like my new look?" I threw my arms around him and he gave me a bear hug anyway. I had changed all right and I wasn't going back.

During my time with the first show, Mom had been busy, too. She loved me and missed me, but she knew I wasn't happy and that I was too pigheaded to come home.

She decided to take a risk. There was a traveling show playing in Portland and they had gotten a very good review. Mom's interest had been aroused when the article mentioned the dancers that could "really dance." Mom decided to call the star of the show and ask him a couple of questions. A couple of questions led to a few more, and before I knew it he was flying us to Las Vegas for an audition. Actually, Mom paid her own way. I loved the dance routines, the people, the atmosphere, everything. This was the kind of dancing I had studied for. This was hot, this was it. He offered me a job.

The only problem was that I already had a job and it's difficult to leave a show when all your costumes have been designed around your body, you know the numbers, and no one else would want the job you are desperate to leave. I gave my resignation and the leader of the show was livid.

"You can't just leave!" he yelled at me.

"I'll give you two weeks to replace me." I was scared and uncertain.

I learned just how egomaniacal everyone was when no one but the light guy was happy for me. The show wasn't working, no one was happy, but no one was willing to rise above it either. I couldn't wait to get out of there.

They brought another girl in but she couldn't hack it. No one else wanted the job or they didn't try very hard to find someone, and when it came time for me to leave, I couldn't. I suppose I could have just walked out on the show and ruined the group, but that's not the kind of person I am. I gave up the new job and stayed in a bad situation. I was miserable and Terry, the producer and star of the other show, was incredulous.

"How can you stay with a show that doesn't work for you? he asked me over the phone from the East Coast.

"I made a commitment and I can't leave these people in the lurch," I said, but I knew I was a stupid fool to ruin this chance by staying to help a group of people who couldn't care less about me or my future. "You should understand perfectly, because I wouldn't do it to you either."

I'd like to say I made the decision because I have such strong morals and fortitude. Actually, I was foolish enough to believe that there would be opportunities like this around every corner. There is something wonderful about being young and ignorant.

What could he say to my logic? The new show hired another dancer and I went on singing and hardly dancing with the show I was with. We continued to travel in a haphazard pattern, seeing the United States and the under-belly of American life. We were in Clarksville, Tennessee, playing at an awful place. The room I was staying in had damp, moldy carpet from the bathroom doorway to the edge of the bed. I had to jump from the bed to the linoleum floor of the bathroom to avoid catching a fungus on my feet.

The next day, our leader gathered us together to pay us and announced in a nonchalant voice, "We don't have a booking for next week, so you all get a week off." He paused to let that information register. "Then we have two weeks in Florida!" he said, like it was a gift.

Things didn't seem right. We were currently in Tennessee, we had no job or income for a week and then we needed to be in Florida? How would we get there? Who would pay for next week's rooms? If we went home, how would we get to Florida from Oregon? The answer? We were on our own.

There I was, in the middle of nowhere, with no money and no place to go for a week. If I used the credit card my dad had given me I would owe my parents the money for the flight home and then one to Florida. I was already constantly in debt, even though I worked like a dog. All the group members were making plans, and none of them included me.

I discovered that the light man, Mark, was going to drive the equipment truck to Pennsylvania and stay at his sister's for the week and then drive the truck down to

Florida. He said I could come if I wanted. I made a call and as luck would have it the show I had auditioned for still needed a dancer, and they were playing just outside of Pittsburgh. I took a risk and hitched a ride with Mark to Pennsylvania.

Traveling to Pittsburgh turned out to be the best move I could have made, because it led to a second chance with the new show. This time, I took the opportunity. It was tough going at first and the band I left was not happy with me, but I knew I had to pick up and get going. Originally I was only going to rehearse with the new show for a week and then continue down to Florida with Mark. But as soon as he saw what I could do, Terry rushed me into a performance. When Mark saw how much the show fit me, he told me he would no longer give me a ride to Florida, and that I would be a fool to give up this opportunity. He said just the right thing, and I stayed. Sometimes it's the risks you don't take that are your biggest mistakes. I'm glad I didn't know any better; I've been trying to do it that way ever since.

Pickup #23: Take the risk so you never have to wonder.

Had I not risked asking my teacher for help, not risked going on the road, and not risked hitching a ride to Pennsylvania, I wouldn't have ended up doing the dance I was supposed to do.

Pickup #24: When risks don't work out, don't make the same mistake twice.

I took a risk and stayed with the original band in the beginning and that taught me a lesson. Even though my personal integrity was sound, I could not live my life well with people who don't share my values or goals. I didn't belong in the first group and staying with it was a poor decision. I'm glad God gave us that one-week opening, so I could get up and get going on continuing my dream.

Pickup #25: Keep on asking yourself, "Is this all there is?"

Before I left home I knew there was more to life than I'd experienced so far. When I was with the first band I kept asking myself, "Is this all there is?" The answer pushed me into another group. Now as a writer and speaker, I'm continually moving past the knowledge I've attained. When we ask ourselves, "Is this all there is?" the answer is always, "No, there's more." Practicing this routine helps us get up and go get it!

Pickup #26: Be curious.

I wanted to travel so I could perform, but also so I could see new places, meet different kinds of people and learn things I didn't know. If we want motivation all we have to do is be curious. Ask questions, go around the next corner, be open to new experiences and grow. Children are full of curiosity and seem to have unlimited energy; learn to be as curious as a kid and watch what happens!

So...

Take the risk so you never have to wonder.

When risks don't work out, don't make the same mistake twice.

Keep on asking yourself, "Is this all there is?"

Be curious.

8

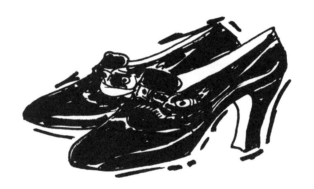

Stay on Balance

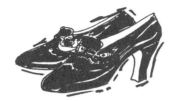

Stay on
Balance

Fall seven times, stand up eight.
—Japanese Proverb

I was sick, and being sick in Las Vegas is no fun. My body was sweating and freezing at the same time and I had big goose bumps all over. I didn't smell very good either: I had the pungent, sour smell that comes out of your pores when the flu bug has you in its grip. My skin was a pasty white, which made the stage makeup I was wearing stand out on my face in a garish and comical way. Staring at myself in the mirror before the show was like looking at someone I didn't know. There was a faint resemblance, like that of a distant cousin maybe, or somebody's great-grandchild; but other than the familiar nose, jutting chin and high forehead, I didn't look like myself at all.

My eyes were sunken and glazed over; my skin was sallow and there were traces of bruising around one eye. The hot-roller frying and the half a can of hair spray I had inflicted on my hair had not helped. It hung in limp, dingy curls, and clung close to my throbbing skull. What was I doing in this costume and how could I possibly perform?

Claudia, my dance partner, gave me a forced smile. "You'll be OK." She patted my clammy and goose-bumpy arm. "We'll just take it easy tonight."

This girl didn't know the word easy. She was short, dark and wired, and she had choreographed both shows, possibly to prove just how much energy and stamina she had. There just isn't any way to do a Russian Cossack dance, a four-minute cancan with flying splits and two-person mounts, a tap routine and three jazz numbers easily. Not to mention the soft shoe number in the cookie monster costume. I smiled weakly, unable to say anything.

Perhaps our boss, the star of the show, would take pity on me and not call us out as often to perform. No such luck. The music started and we ran out to the beat of the drum, the blare of the horns, the frenzy of the bass and electric guitar and the shock of several dozen spotlights blinding our eyes. I followed Claudia on stage and somehow summoned the energy I needed to make my feet move.

We made it through the first number and I stumbled off stage as sickness overtook me. Claudia had an ice bucket backstage which came in handy as I lost what little dinner I had in my stomach. I briefly felt better so I changed into the next costume. We usually performed seven or eight dance numbers in each forty-five minute show, sometimes changing costumes in less than two minutes. Changing fast is an acquired skill and an entire production in itself. You must analyze and prepare, have a system, and work at combining tasks to save time. I was happy that a system was in place.

The next dance number was a spoof on gangsters. We dressed in old-fashioned, oversized suits, with spats, hats and white gloves, and we wore fake black mustaches secured to the front of our powdered upper lips with black electrical tape. Tonight my lip wasn't powdered, it was shiny with tiny sweat beads, and no matter how hard I pressed the mustache on, it peeled slowly from my lip. The mustache had a little clip that gripped on the underside of my nose, fastening on that little piece of cartilage between the nostrils, but the tape really was the stabilizing force, except for tonight.

I went on-stage with a lopsided mustache hanging over my mouth and a fake cigar in my hand. This number was easier because I didn't have to smile. After I fumbled my way through the number, my head went into the ice bucket again as I got rid of lunch. Still the music played and we changed costumes quickly. When it came time for the cancan, my body was so spent from losing my guts in the ice bucket, and I was so stricken with the shakes, that I ran out onto the stage like a woman possessed. I just had to make it through this number. Come on, Shawna! You can do it! I urged myself on. I twirled instead of cart wheeled, I shook my skirt harder instead of kicking like normal. When it came time to grab Claudia around the waist for the two-person mount I clutched her as hard as I could and heard her yell, "Come on Schuhzie!" I grabbed the inside of my foot and hoisted that leg up and around we went, with Claudia doing most of the work and me hanging on for dear life and not dropping my leg for anything.

My head went into the ice bucket again after that number. Then, as the selections wheeled by in a sickening daze, I could cough up nothing into the ice bucket—dry heaves. After the show, I staggered up the spiral staircase to the dressing rooms and sank down onto the floor. I was freezing cold and my teeth began to clatter as Claudia piled coats and costumes on top of me to keep me warm. I let Claudia do the tear down and I don't know how I got home.

I was living with my Aunt Lee at the time and she was completely out of her element coping with my flu. She didn't know what to do with a sick, ultra-thin dancer who couldn't break her fever or keep anything down. Thank heavens the next day was an off day and I could sleep.

I could have, that is, if Aunt Lee would have quit waking me up to check on me. I knew she was concerned about how bad I looked, but each time I began to drift off into some healing sleep, she would push the bedroom door open and tiptoe in, followed by one of her four small dogs, who would jump up onto the bed and jostle me awake.

My aunt's dogs were her pride and joy. She spoiled those little yappers beyond belief, which showed what a soft heart she had. They delighted in waking me up and making my misery worse. As soon as they jumped up onto the bed, my aunt chastised them in a loud, and obviously feigned, stern voice, which pounded in my ears and thundered around my throbbing head. I needed sleep and I needed to be left alone. I had already endured more than I could take.

All the fortitude I had was being stretched to the limit by the unfortunate stream of events that had been occurring lately in my life. It was as if I had signed up for a term of Hardship 101.

Just two weeks before, Claudia and I had gone to take a master dance class from a hot choreographer in town. We traveled out to a studio quite a ways from the Las Vegas strip, dropped our bags against the back wall and started to warm up. The place was packed with some of the best dancers in town, men and women from the Tropicana, the Flamingo Hilton and every other show playing in Vegas. Lean, tight bodies were bending and stretching as we found a place at the barre to join in. The choreographer was known for his incredible kicks and turns. He had been an ice skater in another traveling show and his balance was awesome. His turns were like a spinning top; fascinating and powerful. During the class, he put us through our paces in a rapid-fire manner, constantly changing the combinations and steps to push us harder and to incorporate more style.

After the warm-up, the instructor had us break into two groups and directed each group to line up against a side wall. Then one at a time, each dancer stepped out across the floor from the back corner, doing the latest combination in a diagonal direction to end in the farthest front corner. From that position a different dancer on the other side of the room sprang out from the back corner and traversed the room. In this fashion each dancer crossed the room without colliding with another dancer. The room was large and there were mirrors from floor to ceiling against the front wall, which we faced.

The pressure on each performer was intense because all the other dancers watched and judged as each individual, aware of the critical eyes on her, took her turn. The instructor was completely in charge and he kept making the moves more rapid and difficult. We needed to pay attention as he changed the combination of moves. I was having the time of my life! The music was great, I was stretching myself past where I'd been before and I was feeling good.

About halfway through the class, the instructor changed the combination to a great kick and turn routine with a step out, high kick, body roll down over your leg with a final head snap at the end of the body roll. Then, we had to gather ourselves up to do a double outside turn. Wow! When my turn came, I stepped out and kicked. My leg shot up next to my face and I started the body roll before my foot even touched the floor. The body roll demanded using my torso in a ripple effect with a head snap at the bottom and then up quick, suck in and turn, turn, and step out to repeat. I was sailing!

Claudia was two dancers ahead of me and had just finished her turn as I was beginning mine and I secretly hoped she was watching, because this combination was made for me. I kept building momentum as I kicked and turned and urged myself on to put more power into the kick. I shot my leg up again and again and felt it brush my face. Sometimes in the cancan number, we would get lipstick on our shins from the high kicks, so I usually aimed my leg to pass by the side of my face, which still gave the illusion of a full front kick.

As my leg came down, I started the body roll with incredible energy and force. I love to dance and it felt great to be moving and turning to the music that day. When it came time for the head snap I extended my head back as far as it would go to get a better snap and my effort threw my balance off just a fraction.

What happened next was a big surprise. As I snapped my head forward my forehead somehow collided sharply with my knee and I heard a crack! Whoa! What happened? I came up as fast as I could to finish the combination, but my equilibrium was altered and I was blinded by the hair in my eyes. I staggered toward the mirror as Claudia reached me.

The instructor began to change the combination again so all attention turned to him as I kept running my hand through my hair to remove the strands that were blocking my sight. Then I realized there wasn't any hair blocking my sight. My fingers discovered that my eye was quickly growing shut and I suddenly remembered that I had my contact lenses in. Shock combined with horror as I looked into the mirror and saw my rapidly swelling eye. Claudia was at my side in a moment and propelled me to the bathroom. We pried my left eye open and removed the contact lens.

I didn't finish the class that day. Instead, Claudia drove me to her apartment, the biggest dive in Vegas. We used to joke, wondering how anybody could name an apartment complex Dream World, located on Paradise Avenue. Of course, there is no accounting for taste in Las Vegas.

The whole way home I agonized over the horrible turn of events. "He's gonna kill me!" I kept saying over and over. Our boss was the kind of person who came unglued at the smallest mishap, and here I was with a large one. When I joined his show I had signed a contract that forbade any dangerous activities. If one person in the show got hurt it could put the entire group out of work.

"He's gonna kill me!" I repeated, hoping to gain some sympathy from Claudia.

"Yeah, he is." Claudia affirmed. She was a master at making me feel better.

"What should I do?" I glanced again at my reflection in the mirror. I resembled the Elephant Man.

A heavy thump on the table in front of me signified that Claudia had placed her bag of stage makeup on the table. Combining all the makeup I had, we got to work. We did a pretty decent job, too. With heavy pancake makeup on the skin around my eye and over my brow and nose, and a deep purple eye shadow on the other eye to match the bruised one, I looked like the Elephant Man's distant cousin, more than the Elephant Man himself. The swelling was still a problem and our show was only two hours away. I cringed at the thought of facing Terry, the star and owner of the show. He was a volatile man with a large ego and a grandiose personality. He played at being a big man around town, though in reality he was pretty small potatoes in the Vegas scheme of things. I'd known him to come unglued over some of the smallest things. Once, when I first joined the show, replacing a girl who had been with him from the beginning, I came up with a plan to exchange the shoe boxes that we used to store our costume accessories for tackle boxes that would be better organized and give more protection during travel.

Great idea on my part, but I chose a poor time to suggest it. We were just getting ready to go on stage and Terry was all keyed up. I didn't yet know how excited and tight he got just before a show and I had no idea about his drinking problem. He was standing right inside the curtain before the band started when I decided to confront him with some changes I wanted to make.

"What?" He glared at me as if I were speaking a different language.

"I thought we could upgrade the accessory boxes—" I began. He cut me short. "Those boxes have been used exactly like that since I started this show!" he thundered over the music which had just started when he began to speak.

"Well that doesn't mean they're the best," I cheerfully yelled back over the roar of the drums, which were located next to the curtain we were standing behind. There wasn't enough time to say anything else, because his cue came up and out he went for the first number.

During the show, he ran backstage to change a few things and put on different hats for different numbers. When he came back the first time for a spoof on Nelson Eddy, he was in a mood that was hard for my inexperienced, countrified eyes to believe. He stormed into the dressing room with a vengeance and violence I had never seen and didn't expect. With eyes blazing and sweat pouring down his face, he proceeded to berate me about how things were done in his show and that we would always do it his way. His voice was a high-pitched blast and even with the band playing I was certain they could hear him yelling at me all the way back home.

"My way! It's my show and we'll do it my way!" As he screamed at me, he smacked the back of his hand against my accessory box, shooting it across the dressing room floor. My stuff went flying as the box hit the wall and the contents scattered. Like most things, he had timed his tantrum perfectly and he stomped back on-stage to do his next number as I scrambled to put my box and emotions back together and get ready for my next dance.

I was horrified and couldn't believe the violence he had just shown. With shaking hands I got everything in the box and somewhat in order before racing out for another number. The evening got more frenzied as the show progressed because my stuff was jumbled and I was struggling to control my emotions and get dressed. Besides, I was new to this show and I was out of my element.

Terry had one more costume change during the show and backstage he came again. At nineteen years of age, this whole situation seemed terrifying to me, so I turned my back on him as he grabbed his stuff and demanded some help. I obliged but kept my eyes averted and my body stiff, which must have angered him again, because without a word he struck out with his hand again, knocking my just repacked accessory box against the back wall of the dressing room for the second time that night.

We were almost finished with the show and somehow I made it through the last number. When the music stopped at the end of the show, I listened as if my life depended on it for his footsteps on the dance floor leading to our dressing area. He didn't return, and I didn't cry, but my lip was bleeding from biting down on it as I carefully replaced everything in my now tattered and torn accessory box.

"I probably wouldn't talk to him just before a show again," Claudia needlessly counseled me as she packed up her stuff to leave. She was living with the light man, who also did a karate act, and they hung out together after the show, which left me totally alone, at nineteen years old, on the road with a maniac.

Persevering in a situation like that took all the courage I had, but it had taken a lot of gumption for me to go on the road in the first place. I was getting used to being on the edge and out of control. I was developing toughness and fortitude, whether I wanted to or not.

As Claudia and I sat staring at my puffed eye reflection with two hours to go before the show, I couldn't imagine the reaction I would receive from Terry. I was thankful that Claudia and I were now friends, so that I had an ally. I was also thankful that I had been with the show long enough to gauge Terry's moods and mannerisms and save myself lots of grief. I had certainly learned some great skills during my time on the road. The criticism we endured and the abuse we suffered make me roar with laughter now. But it was serious back then and I could very well have lost my job over the black eye incident.

I didn't want it all to end over a stupid little black eye, a small event in the long list of trials I experienced during my five years on the road. I went to work that night deciding to act nonchalant, as though people popped themselves in the eye all the time. What of it? But I was quaking in my shoes.

I didn't lose my job. I did get chastised in front of the entire troupe, which didn't seem as bad as times before. I was either getting used to the yelling or my boss was getting softer on me. I'm sure it wasn't the latter. He even blamed Claudia for not watching out for me. Of course, all our dance class privileges were taken away. I remember his parting words as we were about to go on for the show. "For heaven's sake, Shawna, keep your bad side away from the audience!" I remember thinking how much I appreciated his concern.

The silver lining in the black cloud of having a black eye was that it forced me to improve my makeup skills. My injured eye started out a vibrant purple and blue combination and slowly evolved into a tropical yellow and green look that was easier to match with makeup but looked horrid with my costumes.

The eye was not healed and still showed signs of bruising as I lay in my room at my aunt's with the flu. It had been an eventful couple of weeks, that was for sure! With no makeup on, a faded black eye and the pallor from being sick, I wasn't a pretty sight and I saw the worry in my aunt's eyes.

"Aunt Lee?" I reached for her hand. Mercifully she had come in without the dogs. Aunt Lee was a big, strong, intimidating woman, who wore her hair short in a masculine cut and carried herself like an army sergeant. She had been the first female pit boss in Las Vegas and she had fought like the dickens to get where she was. She had given up a lot to be successful and had no children of her own. She came across rough and tough and could be a pretty hard cookie. Only I knew that she had a soft and gooey center.

"What, baby?" she whispered.

"I know this doesn't look good right now—" I started.

"Oh, you don't look so bad!" she said in her gruff and abrupt way.

"Anyway," I continued, "I'm already feeling better, but I really, really, really need to sleep for awhile and I know you won't let anyone disturb me, OK?" I gave her the best smile I could muster.

"OK, baby." She got up from the side of the bed. "Leave it to me." Finally she had something to be in charge of, something to do. I rolled over and fell asleep at last.

It's easier to sleep when you know you can overcome things. When you know you possess the fortitude it takes to get up and keep going. The power comes from your mind, and your belief system. The black eye and the time when Terry had showed me his violent streak helped me to be strong. I can't say I recommend the way some of the lessons were administered, but I'm glad I made it through. I don't remember ever being as sick as I was while I dragged myself on stage, or as scared, or as naive. I am, however, still great at makeup application, speaking my mind at the wrong time, and throwing myself off balance. It's a good thing I had skills, since soon I would find myself out of a job.

Pickup #27: Have a system in place for getting through upsetting times.

Without a system for dressing rapidly, I could not have gone on with the show during my sickness. Each time we take the time to develop systems we give ourselves a little advantage. Doing something the practiced way, or developing good habits, gives you something to fall back on, something to hold on to. From paying your bills, to exercise, set up a system and it will be easier to get up on down days.

Pickup #28: Pick the right time to suggest changes and ideas.

Learn when to suggest changes and when to offer ideas. It's up to us to learn to gauge another's mood before we speak. I learned the hard way when to speak and when to hold my tongue, but it's worked to my benefit ever since. I'm very rarely deterred when I have an idea or want to make a change because I watch and listen for the best time to speak.

Pickup #29: Learn to be alone.

I grew up when I learned I could get through bad times alone. You have everything you need no matter where you find yourself or what situation you're in. The road was a lonely place, but it helped me understand that true motivation is about internal fortitude and not what others give or take away from you.

Pickup #30: Pull yourself up and face the music.

I was in trouble after I whacked myself in the eye. I knew it, I couldn't get out of it, and so I pulled myself up and kept on going. When you make a mistake or an accident happens, pull yourself up, learn what there is to learn and put the past behind you. It really doesn't matter what has gone on before, move forward and you'll feel better.

So...

Have a system in place for getting through
upsetting times.

Pick the right time to suggest changes and
ideas.

Learn to be alone.

Pull yourself up and face the music.

9

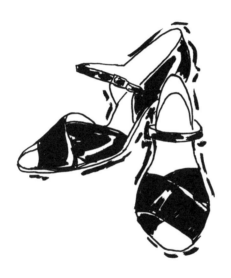

Keep Your Faith

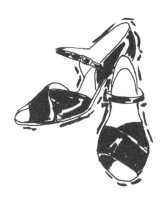

Keep Your
Faith

*Faith is raising the sail of our little boat until it
is caught up in the soft winds above and picks up
speed, not from anything within itself, but from the
vast resources of the universe around us.*
—W. Ralph Ward, Jr.

I knew I could get a job. I didn't know how, but I had faith
that a job would come my way. In the meantime, I audi-
tioned every chance I got. Auditions were held at dance
studios and there was time to warm up and stretch out
before you performed. Most auditions had great routines
that tested your abilities and gave you a great workout too.
Auditions were conducted for specific shows, but I was
open for anything. The tryout system wasn't a bad way to
stay in shape, and you could discover how you fit in among
the company of other unemployed dancers who were
seeking work. I was living with my Aunt Lee in Las Vegas
again, after a short, unsuccessful attempt to move back to
Oregon and live at home. Without a job, I couldn't afford to

pay for regular dance classes so auditions were one way to learn and stay in shape.

I had left my parents' house, with all my worldly possessions piled in the back of my car. Good thing I didn't own much. My aunt gave me free room and board and the Las Vegas sun was good for my spirits and great for my tan.

I didn't want to work for a big show and become a Vegas dancer. That didn't interest me and I refused to go topless. Not that anyone would have wanted me topless. I was pretty thin and not at all top heavy.

I had decided on Vegas out of blind faith. Many dancers hung out in the desert city, because dozens of shows were put together there. I would find a place in the entertainment industry, I just knew it.

I learned of an audition for dancers to join a European tour and that fascinated me. I had never been to Europe and thought it might be fun. The men doing the audition were dressed very well and the routines were punchy and fast. I liked the feel of the situation immediately. When my turn came, I did very well, but I knew performance alone was not enough. In dancing, as in acting, many people could do the same job; ultimately the decision is based on a dancer's appearance, height and hair color. In order to stand out among the many talented people competing, you must continue to demonstrate your skills, pray, and see what happens. If I didn't get the European tour job, I knew I'd get something else.

After the audition, while people were still milling around, I had just removed my shoes, the tall, silver, show-dancing kind—when the head of the show called me over.

"My, you are a short one aren't you!" he said as I stood next to him, eye to eye, in my bare feet. I was thinking to myself how similar in height we were as I raised up on my toes in defense.

"How tall are you, dear?" he asked in a patronizing voice.

"How tall do you need?" came my cocky reply.

His laughter was more like a squeal. "Weeellllll, we have a live one here don't we?" he said to no one in particular. "You just might do very well. Would you like to join us in Europe?"

"When do we leave?" I had myself a job.

I had been in Las Vegas for only two weeks when I packed my car again, kissed Aunt Lee good-bye and headed home to Oregon once again, to put my belongings in storage for the duration of the European tour. I had signed a six-month contract to travel with the show throughout Europe, with an additional month of rehearsals, so I knew I would be gone seven months at the very least. I was young and determined and had absolutely nothing to tie me down. I figured if I liked the strange land across the Atlantic, I might never come home.

Details fell into place quickly and I left for the airport and my first stop in Los Angeles with one brimming bag and my international electrical converter. I knew absolutely no one who was going to be in the troupe. My instructions were to meet a man at the Los Angeles airport, who would be holding a sign with my name printed on it.

Richard was tall and fair, with a mustache and sandy blond hair. He was the costume designer and would be meeting up with the show in Portugal. Until then, he was my stopover in Los Angeles. He fed me, gave me his bed to sleep in and acted oblivious to the fact that I wasn't even smart enough to be frightened. The international flight he put me on the next morning was a jumble of customs checks and passport information; I was a blind and silly girl who trusted everyone. God must have assigned an angel exclusively to watch over me, because I arrived in Portugal without losing my life or my luggage.

The dancers were arriving in Portugal from points all over, only three of us from the United States. I guess the producers felt compelled to include at least a few Americans in the cast, since the show was called "All-American Girls."

Most of the girls were from England, Canada, and Spain. We were housed in hotels and were immediately placed into extreme rehearsals, which left us feeling exhausted and wrung out. I learned, first hand, the difficulty of living in a country where you do not speak or understand the language, where you have no friends, and where everyone is in some form of competition.

Dancers are competitive. Each of us wanted the best spot, the most featured dances and the title of dance captain, which paid more and held more prestige. Because the show was new, all the positions were up for grabs. There were a few girls who had worked for the producer before and knew the ropes, but most of us were in the dark. I was amazed and appalled to learn that some of the women had been performing in shows since they were sixteen years old. What had happened to their schooling? What would they do next? I also learned that even though we were all considered to be dancers, there was a very strong distinction between "dancers" and "walkers."

The "dancers" danced. We did the hard stuff, the grueling stuff, the moves that brought the sweat out. The "walkers" were the tall and beautiful girls who slinked and strutted and demonstrated how beautiful the female form could be. The walkers were topless and the audience was enthusiastic about their bareness. We dancers added excitement, stayed covered, but had costuming that was alluring and mysteriously feminine.

There was one walker who had been in these productions all of her life. Her name was Gayle and she was a stunning, six-foot beauty with flaming red hair and a chest that would make a celibate sit up and notice. Because of her height and magnificence, she commanded center stage and strutted her stuff better than most. She was angling for the dance captain role and made no bones about the fact that it should be hers. I knew I was a far superior dancer and also had more skill in human relations, but I was frightened to speak up and ask for the opportunity to compete.

I was so far out of my element that it's difficult to describe. Place yourself in another country, unable to speak the language. Mix in a cosmopolitan group of people from all regions of the world with different backgrounds and ages. Stir in the sexual equation and potential intimacy between producers, managers, dancers, and wardrobe people, and place into this milieu a young, impressionable country girl. Strange and daring ideas, costumes and temptations flooded my head. Exotic music, gambling and foreign cultural customs became part of an ordinary day. I did my best to keep my head above water and lived through those first days by concentrating totally on the dances, the steps, the moves, the sweat and the routines. I worked hard and I excelled.

Robert, one of two male dancers in the troupe, said to me one day, "Shawna, you need to let them know that you want to be dance captain."

I was pleased that he had noticed me, but I could feel myself getting embarrassed.

"You'd be perfect!" he added. "You're the best dancer in the bunch and you really should be the only one considered."

His attention was flattering and I secretly hoped he was right; but I knew that Gayle was angling for the part and I didn't want to step on any toes. I also feared being turned down.

"I would love to be dance captain, but I can't ask for it." I was intense. "If I'm good enough, they will ask me."

"Shawna, don't be stupid." Robert's voice turned to stone. "In this world, you have to look out for number one, and you have to self-promote." He shook his head at my ignorance.

"Maybe so, Robert, but I'm going to wait and see. I have complete faith that if they want the best dancer, they will pick who deserves the job." I set my jaw.

"OK, if you want to be stubborn. But I know Gayle is asking them for the job right now!" He implored me with his eyes. "Shawna, at least let them know you're interested!"

"I'm sorry, Robert," I said, determined not to advance my case.

"I think you're wrong," he said and walked away.

I've thought about Robert's advice many times, and if I had it all to do over I probably would go to the choreographer and the director and let them know that I was interested in the role. For people to give you what you want, they need to know what you want.

But I was prideful and conceited and I wanted to have them tell me I was good. I wanted to win the job over a woman who willingly removed her top to dance. I may have been part of a topless show, but I had disdain for the women who exposed themselves for a living. Looking back, I guess

I wasn't much different. I wore very suggestive clothing while dancing and even on my time off, but I never allowed my breasts to be my selling point. I had studied dance all my life and I wanted to be judged by my dancing.

I've changed my mind about topless dancers since those days in Europe. I've also changed my mind about a lot of things. I learned that the women who chose to take off their tops were some of the nicest, biggest-hearted people I ever met. They were warm and funny and had high moral standards. Using their assets didn't seem at all strange to them and didn't affect how they lived or treated others. It was not my place to judge anyone; I was wrong to do it then. The difference between the walkers and me wasn't a case of how good or bad we thought ourselves on the outside, it was how we viewed ourselves from the inside.

During a break before rehearsal one afternoon, the assistant to the director knocked on the door to our room. I was sharing quarters with two English dancers and one Canadian. I opened the door to find a young man with slicked-back hair, too much cologne, and expensive clothing encasing his skinny frame.

"Great," he said, "you're just the one I need." He grinned. "The boss wants to see you right away in the rehearsal hall about the dance captain position. Come down as soon as you're ready." He turned on his heel and was gone.

I didn't say a word but as I shut the door I suddenly felt quite dizzy. I wandered into the bathroom and shut the door. Something released inside of me and I staggered to the bidet and vomited all I had eaten that day. It's probably the only time in my life that I have thrown up without being sick or intoxicated. I just needed to rid myself of the worry and the concern. I flushed the bidet and pulled myself together.

When I went down to the showroom, the place was empty and the stage was bare. I absorbed the atmosphere as I noted the richly colored curtains, the plush booths that lined the walls and the shine on the revolving dance floor. Lisbon was the port of kings and dignitaries in past times and I could envision a royal dignitary or two sitting in this luxurious ballroom. Almost hidden by the tall back of one of the chairs sat the producer, Bill. He was so feminine, and the chair dwarfed him and made him appear even smaller than he was. Funny that this little man could put fear into all the people in the show. What a temper he had! I think it has something to do with control. Little people, and by that I mean little in integrity, are the ones to watch out for whenever they come into a position of power. I sat down tentatively.

"We're going to make you dance captain, Shawna." He used the plural even though only he and I were sitting there and I knew it was his decision alone.

"I won't let you down," I said humbly.

"I know," he replied with a smile. "That's why I am taking a chance with you. You make fifty extra a week and don't let those girls run over you."

That was it. He dismissed me with a wave of his hand without ever telling me what a dance captain did, should do, or was expected to do. I decided right then that I needed some friends and advice but was being put into a position where I could be an enemy and adversary. More lessons were coming, I could tell.

Pickup #31: Know that opportunities are endless.

I didn't worry too much when I went to Vegas because I had faith that there was a job out there somewhere. That's faith and a hopeful attitude, both excellent things to have if you want to keep your spirits up. I have found, in living my life, that there are always opportunities if you keep on getting up, getting going and looking for them.

Pickup #32: Stay focused.

When placed in a situation that was uncomfortable and unusual I survived by focusing on the task at hand. I worked on the dance, the moves, the routines, and that kept me from drowning in worry about the things I couldn't control. There are always things that can upset us. Focus on the things you can do and that will help you keep on moving.

Pickup #33: Ask for what you want.

Jesus said, "Ask and you shall receive." If you wait for someone else to give you what you want you may never get it. I was foolish not to ask to be the dance captain and though it turned out all right, I felt like someone who narrowly misses having an accident, more aware and smarter for the experience. Now I ask for what I want and it's a great motivator since what we ask for we usually feel responsible for.

Pickup #34: Keep your faith.

Faith is a hard concept because you can't see it, or touch it. You can feel it, however, in yourself and in others. Through the centuries people have sustained themselves with faith. When you don't know what you are doing or where you are going, keep your faith and truly, things will work out. As you see things in your mind, so they become in reality.

So...

Know that opportunities are endless.

Stay focused.

Ask for what you want.

Keep your faith.

10

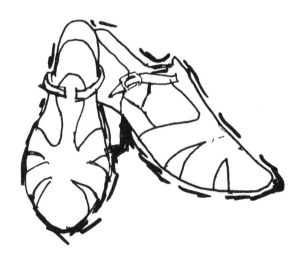

Be Persistent

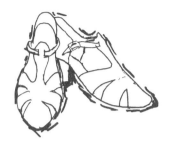

Be Persistent

Persistence is what makes the impossible possible, the possible, likely, and the likely definite.
—Robert Half

"Hi, this is Shawna Schuh, are there any auditions coming up?" I asked excitedly into the phone.

"Who is this again?" replied a tired female voice.

"This is Shawna Schuh, and I'm new with the agency and I was told to call this number to inquire about upcoming auditions; are there any?" There was silence on the other end of the line which I felt compelled to fill: "Am I calling the right number? Am I doing it right?"

"Yes, you have the right number and no, there aren't any auditions."

"OK, thank you." I hung up the phone. I fought back disappointment; what did I expect the first time I called? An audition for a movie with Mel Gibson? I waited and called back the next day.

"Hi, this is Shawna Schuh, is anything up?" I had expectancy in my voice.

"No, nothing, Shawna," came the weary reply. It must be a lot of work dealing with unemployed actors all day.

My goal was to call every day so that the actor's agency wouldn't forget me, and to stop by the office every so often so that the people there would have my face in their minds. I swung by the agency every time I could when I looked especially nice and hung out with all the other actors and models who were doing the same thing. I picked up quite a bit of information and the lingo of the business in my sporadic stop-bys. Most of the actors talked about recent auditions, in which the directors "loved" them, or bad auditions in which they weren't "right" for the part. The whole thing, the conversations, the hopes, dreams, disappointments and successes were very exciting.

"Hi, this is Shawna Schuh, is anything up?" I asked again. I had been calling the agency every day for three months and by now I was really using my acting skills. Every day, though, I got the same answer, "No, nothing, Shawna."

I was beginning to doubt myself. I hadn't been sent out on a single audition. How would they know whether I could act if I wasn't given a chance to show my stuff? I started to read self-help books, I went to see motivation expert Zig Ziglar. He said to "expect the best," so I did. Nothing happened.

"Hi, this is Shawna Schuh. Are there any auditions on the horizon?" Sometimes I'd alter my question hoping the answer would be different. It wasn't. By the fourth month I was thinking about quitting. Who was I anyway to think that I could act? I was a dancer. Where did I get off dreaming that someone would hire me, anyway? My spirits sank lower, but I continued to call every day.

"Hi, anything up for Shawna Schuh?"

"No, not today, Shawna." Was there a hint of pity in her voice?

"OK, thank you." I got off the phone and sobbed.

"I'm never gonna make it in this business," I thought to myself. So I read more books. I pored over accounts of people overcoming obstacles. There was President Lincoln and all the demeaning failures he endured before finally winning the White House. I repeated affirmations and took more classes in acting, dance and voice. I may not have been getting any work, but I was determined to keep working. I called every day.

"Hi, it's Shawna Schuh wondering if there's anything up?" I acted cheery and up. Once again, rejection.

One day I called as usual with my, "Hi, this is Shawna..." routine, except this time the woman on the other end of the line said, "Hold on a minute, Shawna."

My breath stopped. As I waited on the phone, I heard her take the receiver and place it against her shoulder to muffle the sound, like you do when you yell at the dog to shut up while you're having a conversation. Then I heard the receptionist say in an agitated voice to someone in the office, "Isn't there anything we can send this girl on?"

I wasn't crushed. I was hopeful. My persistence had paid off, she wanted me off her back enough to do something. She returned to the line a couple of minutes later. "Shawna, I have a booking for you!"

A booking! That means a paid job and I hadn't even auditioned yet! This was going to be a great day!

"What job?" I asked, out of breath.

"You're going to be an extra for Fred Meyer!" She sounded very triumphant.

An extra for Fred Meyer. Wow.

In the entertainment business, on a scale of one to ten, with ten being the highest, a job as an extra falls around minus one. An extra is a peon in the acting business, the lowest of the low. Extras are the scenery, the crowd, the legs at a dinner table—they are truly extra. Being an extra is not the kind of job you brag about to anyone, but it was the beginning for me, and I was thrilled.

"So, what part am I playing?" I wanted to cover all the details and get into character. If you know anything about Fred Meyer you know it's a grocery store. Nevertheless, I wanted to know my part. I wanted to start my acting career the most professional way possible.

"You're going to be a shopper." She was smiling at me over the phone, I could tell. She gave me the information rapidly. She told me where to go and what to do and I hung up the phone. An extra for Fred Meyer, and I didn't even have to audition, what a lucky girl I was.

Having been on the road working at various jobs, I knew I didn't want to make a bad first impression on the head man, Jim Card. I didn't really know what to wear, because the location where we were shooting the commercial was a grocery store. A shopper could wear business clothes or flip flops and a tank top. I decided to dress up a little. I wore a crisp shirt and slacks, walking shoes and a blazer, and I carried a shoulder bag. I agonized over this selection for days and finally decided it was better to be overprepared than underprepared. I took some additional clothing items, just in case, and threw everything in my car. OK, I took everything I owned—and borrowed some stuff too.

When I got to the store where we were doing the filming, I was scared out of my wits. I'm always frightened before I do something new. I like the tingly feeling; it reminds me that I am totally alive. It also forces me to be prepared.

I asked for Mr. Card when I arrived and was directed to a short, attractive man with thin blond hair. I summoned all my courage and confidence and said, "Hello, Mr. Card, my name is Shawna Schuh; I'm here to be an extra. I wore what I thought would be appropriate, but I did bring some other choices." I took a deep breath to calm myself, fully expecting him to tell me to go stand in the back.

He took one look at me and said, "Great! I'd like to see what you brought."

"You would?" I scrambled not to show my surprise. I wanted to repeat the part about being an extra, just in case he misunderstood.

"I'm scenery!" I wanted to shout. Instead I silently took him over to where I had dropped off the two bulging hanging bags and extra large duffel bag filled with shoes. He was teaching me a very big lesson right then. Even though I knew that being an extra was a peon job and that no one gave it any respect, he was showing me that the job was important enough that it mattered what I wore. I was the one who thought being an extra was a peon job; in reality, it was just as important to the overall commercial as the lead, just different. I made a vow never again to discount a task I was given. If they were paying me, they expected my best. My goal from that day on was to always do my best, no matter what part I played.

I unzipped my bulging bags to let him see everything I owned. He turned to his assistant and said, "Can you believe this?"

"No, I can't," she replied.

He changed the blazer I had on and my shoulder bag, and had me put my hair behind my ears. I did as I was told, listened to all directions and made it through the shoot without damaging myself or any equipment with my nervousness.

One week later my agent called me. Whoa! Hold the phone, my agent calling me? I didn't know who it was at first.

"Hi Shawna, this is Sam." She sounded pleasant.

"Who is it?" I asked.

"Sam," she replied, "your agent."

"Oh, hi." I had never spoken to her before and didn't know what to say. I needn't have worried; I've learned since that she's never at a loss for words.

"Shawna," she began, "what did you *do* on that job at Fred Meyer?"

Suddenly I felt apprehensive.

"Nothing...why?" I asked in a little voice. Here I was with my first acting job ever and I'd obviously done something wrong or my agent wouldn't be calling me and asking me questions.

"Well," she said in a somewhat incredulous tone, "they just called to book you again, only this time you'll be the non-speaking lead!"

Now I'd like to think it was because I was such a talented extra...

I believe I am talented, but that wasn't what got me re-booked for Fred Meyer. It was being totally prepared and willing to work.

I've come to believe that each and every person born on this earth is talented. Your true job in life is figuring out what your unique talent is and using it to your fullest ability. It's the hardest job you have to do.

I learned that day that talent will never be enough; you must also be prepared. When you are, things move fast. The best part of this lesson is, I never had to play an extra again, and I've never been unprepared for a job.

Pickup #35: Keep going even when you're discouraged.

To really pick up and get going, take action. Make the phone calls, no matter what the answer is; read books on what you're interested in, to improve your expertise; listen to self-help and motivational materials; go see a professional speaker who will lift your spirits and give you some ideas. We all have a choice to either quit or keep going. I think you know by now quitting isn't an option.

Pickup #36: Do your best work, regardless of your position.

I thought being an extra was a peon job, but the man who hired me didn't think so. He was paying me, so he expected my best. It doesn't matter what position we work or play, each position is important in the big scheme of things. Don't discount what you do for a living; if you can make any job excellent, you'll be given excellent jobs.

Pickup # 37: Be overprepared for everything.

I packed everything I owned so I wouldn't find myself without what I needed. This little quirk got me a second job and seven years' worth of work and income from that client besides. I'm now known for being overprepared and not only does it impress those I work for, it relieves fears I might otherwise have about not being able to do a good job. Professionals, and those who keep getting up, overprepare.

Pickup # 38: Dress up for others.

My first job in commercials was for a one-stop shopping center, a grocery store. I knew that I could dress down or I could dress up for them and I chose to do what I thought they might like and it worked. Don't dress for your comfort and convenience, dress for all the people who will be looking at you and working for you. If you want to get your spirits up, put on some color and you'll be amazed at how many people smile at you and compliment you, and how quickly you get your pickup, up.

So...

Keep going even when you're discouraged.

Do your best work, regardless of your position.

Be overprepared for everything.

Dress up for others.

11

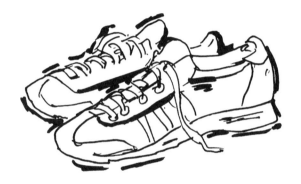

Go with Your Instincts

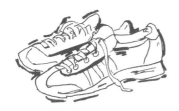

Go with Your Instincts

> *My philosophy is that not only are you respon-*
> *sible for your life, but doing the best at this moment*
> *puts you in the best place for the next moment.*
> —Oprah Winfrey

"Shawna Schuh...you're up next." The voice came drifting out through the darkness.

"Coming," I responded in the most confident voice I could muster.

I had auditioned for a movie and the callbacks were being held at Portland's downtown Red Lion Inn. The production company had taken over an entire wing of the hotel and the callbacks were being conducted in one of the rooms. I had been waiting for my turn in a darkened corner of the parking lot so I wouldn't get freaked out by the other actors and my own emotions.

As I walked briskly forward, I said another quick prayer that God would be with me and that I wouldn't make a fool of myself. The part I was trying out for was pretty important, the female lead in a made-for-cable movie starring Gary Busey. Usually, local actors here in Oregon didn't get to read for any of the good parts. Although the production companies liked to use Portland as a filming location, they set up the stars in Los Angeles and used local talent only for the small, less important roles. I had done several films and always read for the part of the real estate agent, the housewife or someone who was only present in the film to help explain the story.

"Are you ready to read for the part of Marianne?" I was asked as I reached the casting director, a woman in her forties who didn't make time for small talk, especially with actors. She was thin, and had dark brown hair and large, dark glasses perched on her thin and pointed nose. She reminded me of my fourth grade teacher.

"I'm actually ready to read for the part of Susan," I replied and waited. I had originally read for the part of Susan and it was a good scene. When my agent called and told me I had gotten a callback, which is the way this business works, I was thrilled. When she told me it was for Marianne, which was the lead and an even better part, I was even happier. After reading the audition piece for Marianne, I realized that if I read for the part of Susan instead, I would be able to demonstrate a wider range of acting skills. The big question I had was, should I go with my instincts or do what I was told?

"Didn't your agent call you?" the casting director asked me in a tone of voice that registered her annoyance. "Didn't she tell you that you're reading for Marianne?"

"Yes, she did, but I'm more ready to read for Susan." Her displeasure was apparent but I chose to ignore it. This was quite a departure for me and I wasn't going to back down now. You only get to audition for the director once, and only after you've survived one or two elimination auditions with other people. Only five women were left to read for this part. Many times I had jumped in too quickly to read when a part was presented and I didn't do the best I could. I didn't want to blow this opportunity.

Also, it's difficult for a casting director to decide based on only one character or line that the actor has to read, especially if it's something like, "Well, the price does seem somewhat high." Trust me, I've been in some odd auditions.

The most ridiculous audition I remember was when I was trying out for a part as the mother of a young boy whom another woman claimed was hers. In the scene for the audition, the star attempted to take my son from me. Sounds like it could be a great scene, right? Well, my one-word line was "Ken!" as I called out to my husband for support.

That was it! One word! You can imagine how important a person feels when she is called in for a part like that. What is even more incredible is that, based on that one-word line, I got a callback for the part! Back I went to do my one-line reading, this time with a director watching. At least the line was easy to memorize! I really shouldn't make fun, especially since I ended up getting the part and the director was wonderful and gave me more lines to say as the scene was developed.

Having done such small and unimportant auditions in the past made the audition for Susan, with several pages of dialogue, feel like an opportunity to really show the depth of my acting ability. I made up my mind that I was going to read the better audition piece and that was that.

As we entered the audition room, I rubbed my hands down the front of my cords to get the sweat off before I had a seat in front of the director, the producer and a third person, who must have been the director's assistant. The casting director introduced me and added that I was there for the part of Marianne but was reading the Susan part. She mumbled something about my agent and a mix-up. The director, a lean, gray-haired man in his late fifties, smiled at me. All three in the room were dressed in dark colors and seemed relaxed. Of course, why shouldn't they be relaxed? They had nothing to be uptight about, they got to do the choosing!

The casting director sat down next to me and said she would be the one I would read with. She played Gary Busey's part and told me to begin whenever I was ready. I gave myself a moment to calm down and slip into the role. I had worked on it and knew it. I turned to the casting director and she was the only person in the room for me at that moment. I felt myself take focus on the dialogue of my character and we began.

When the scene was over, I took a breath and turned toward the director. He smiled at me again and said, "Very nice work."

They always say something nice even when they hate you.

"I could read the part of Marianne now if you wish." I slipped it out as though it was the most natural thing in the world to be in charge of your own audition.

"Well," he glanced at the producer, a woman in her early forties, who had a great style about her. "We'd love to see it," he said.

After I finished the second scene, he complimented me again as I stood up. I shook his hand, thanked him for the audition and made my way out into the darkness of the parking lot to my car.

When I reached my car and had slipped behind the wheel, I realized my hands were shaking and my body was tingling all over. I pounded my hands on the steering wheel and let out a primal yell. I had done it! I had taken control and performed an audition I was proud of! It didn't matter whether I got the part or not, I was proud of myself. I had been given the opportunity to act, which was my great love anyway; I had found my focus and I had nailed the scenes! I drove home feeling wonderful, totally alive and fully inspired by my act of strength.

I did not hear from my agent. OK, so I didn't do as well as I thought. Maybe they went with a dark-haired woman. In this business it's not always about talent; sometimes you win a part simply because you look like you belong in the family the producer has in mind. I consoled myself with the thought that they had at least asked me to read for the female lead. The part of Marianne was a good role and someone would get a nice paycheck for that part.

I stopped by the modeling school where I worked, and my boss, Chris, called out from her office, "Hey, Shawna! I heard you got a callback for the part of Marianne. Good work!"

"Thanks, Chris." I felt a little strange, because nobody had called me, but I didn't know who had gotten the role. "Who actually got it?" I asked her.

"Probably someone from L.A." She paused to soften the blow. "You know those big parts usually go to a more well-known actor."

"Well, it was fun anyway," I smiled at her. "I thought the audition piece for Susan was stronger to show my range, so I read for both, which was great."

Chris was finished giving me my compliment. "Good for you, Shawna. I'll talk to you later."

I walked down the hall to pick up my paycheck and check the class schedule. I was teaching every week and wanted to see whether any classes had been added. I decided to go over to my agent's office to ask whether anyone had received feedback from the audition. Occasionally the director or casting agent will tell the talent agent why an actor didn't make the cut.

The agency was unusually quiet. Most of the time it was buzzing with actors and models milling around hoping that the phone will ring and the agent will give them the first go. I never felt especially comfortable at the agency; it wasn't like the dance studio, where we performed with each other and everyone knew who was good and who wasn't. In acting, the auditions are always behind closed doors, which leaves the actors to hang around in the halls and waiting areas. Most talk incessantly about themselves and how wonderful they did on their last job.

For some, it's a way to build themselves up before they go in to be judged. I never liked to wait with the other actors, preferring instead to be away and with my own thoughts before an audition. You wouldn't believe how many times someone at the audition would completely freak you out and ruin your chance before you went in to read. That happened to me a couple of times before I realized I needed to focus on the task at hand and not worry about anyone but myself.

On this particular day, I didn't find anyone downstairs except the receptionist, who looked bored as she did some filing. I headed upstairs. My agent was sitting at her desk with piles of papers and pictures around her, when I stuck my head in. "Hi, Nanette!" I called out just loud enough to get her attention.

"Oh hi, Shawna, congratulations!" she smiled at me.

"Thanks, Nanette, the callback was fun," I began. "Did they say anything about my performance?" This is always a sticky question, because your agent doesn't want to tell you anything that will destroy you, but she also doesn't want to imply something positive if nothing was said. I can imagine how hard it is to have actors constantly calling you, stopping by for compliments on auditions, only to have to tell them that nothing at all was mentioned about them. If you want to make people unhappy, be an agent. For every person who gets a key part, many others are disappointed.

"No," she said airily, "only that you got the part."

My mouth dropped. "What part?" My voice was hollow, this was such a shock.

"The part of Marianne, silly, don't tell me you didn't know," she giggled.

"I didn't know." Happiness began to bubble up inside me. "Nobody called me so I thought they went with somebody else."

"Well, now you know," she said. "Congratulations!"

I went bouncing down the stairs and out into the crisp fall air. What a life I lead, I thought, from despair to euphoria in about three seconds flat. The someone who was going to play the female lead was me. I couldn't wait to get started!

Pickup #39: Stick with your instincts.

So many times I've gone against my better judgment and been sorry for it. When I decided to defy the casting agent and go with what felt right for me, I was finally successful. Don't be frightened of what your heart and gut tell you, listen.

Pickup #40: Try new things.

I had never before taken control of one of my auditions and doing so taught me that it's better when you are out front living and experiencing things rather than letting someone else dictate your future. Trying new things adds confidence and courage to your arsenal of knowledge. You can't gain experience and be on the cutting edge if you don't try new things.

Pickup #41: Be ready for the unexpected.

I wasn't too depressed when I thought someone else had gotten the part instead of me, but I was elated when I found out unexpectedly that I had gotten it after all. I have found life to be full of unexpected twists and turns, which make it interesting and keep us all guessing. When you have a good attitude and expect that anything can happen, lots of interesting things do. Be ready to get going no matter what is going on; it's more fun anyway.

So...

Stick with your instincts.

Try new things.

Be ready for the unexpected.

12

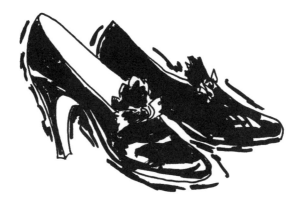

Change Course
if You Need To

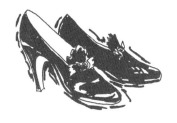

Change Course if You Need To

Calm self-confidence is as far from conceit as the desire to earn a decent living is remote from greed.

—Channing Pollock

Walking onto the set was like walking into the Twilight Zone. A film set is definitely a world of its own. Like a mini city on wheels, everything is portable and can be moved from place to place. Each person is assigned a particular job, which he or she does with the utmost intensity, usually with a walkie-talkie plastered to an ear or mouth. I had been on film sets several times before, but never as the female lead. This wasn't a huge part but in the film business, like any business, everybody feels more comfortable when your status can be defined quickly so that they can treat you accordingly. In previous ventures when I was in a film, I had been a day player and relegated to the "honey wagon," which is where the toilets are located, and the tiny trailer dressing rooms, to which anyone with lines is assigned.

These miniature dressing rooms are pretty sad, in keeping with the diminutive size of your role, but at least you have an honest-to-goodness dressing room. In my first film experience, I was cast as a young bride looking for a home with her husband. The only purpose for this character was to establish that the lead actor, James Garner, was a real estate agent. The shot was of Mr. Garner driving me and my young husband up in his car as if we had been looking at homes and were returning to his office. He helped me out of the car and asked me what I thought of the houses he had just shown us. My big line in this film? "They are a little high."

That was it. That was all I had to say. But those five words put me into the "speaking part" category, which meant I received day-player wages, had a dressing room with my name felt-penned on the front door, and I was mentioned in the film's credits. The actor who played my husband didn't have any lines, which meant he was only an extra. Even though he and I did the same amount of work and were on the set for the same amount of time, no lines for him meant no dressing room, and a lower rate of pay. No one said life was fair and in the entertainment business it never even pretends to be.

My first experience was pretty impressive. Meeting and working with James Garner was an encounter I will never forget. I was only with him for a short time, and he would never remember me, but I still marvel at how professional he was. When he appeared on set to go over the scene with me, I expected Maverick to come riding up, or Rockford to stride out in his hip seventies garb. Instead, this bent-over, crippled older man came out. I was startled by his appearance and his frailty. He was gracious and wonderful, though he didn't extend his hand because of arthritis. When the crew was lighting the scene where, in the script, we part ways in front of his office, two stand-ins came and took our places. Imagine, a stand-in for me when I only had five words! Mr. Garner took my arm and we went over and sat in the tall director chairs you always see on movie sets. His name was emblazoned on the chair he sat in and I sat in the director's chair.

Mr. Garner chatted with the people around him, talking about baseball, I think. I was so awestruck that I said even less than the words given to my film character. When we walked back to our spots and the assistant director yelled, "Quiet on the set!" I saw the biggest transformation occur that I have ever seen. James Garner took a breath and began to pull himself up, up, up and back, making himself bold and incredible. Suddenly before me stood the TV idol of my youth. He was so "on" that he glowed—he was magnificent!

The scene took us about three seconds to do; how could I foul up something that simple? The director yelled, "Cut!" and Mr. Garner began to shrink back to the little old man who was there before the camera rolled. The rest of the time I watched him, he acted in each scene only once and he was a consummate professional every moment. I heard through sources on the set that he was known for doing most shots in one take and never making mistakes. I believed it.

Other small roles followed for me, and I always had lines, which meant I always had a dinky dressing room and was usually treated like a nobody day-player, which I was. On this occasion, however, I was ushered to my own trailer, which was painted on the outside with big letters that read "Star Wagon." Wow! I stepped inside and the producer's assistant (PA) told me to relax and that someone would come and get me when the makeup artist was ready for me. I, of course, had come forty-five minutes early, because I was nervous and scared. After the door was shut, I glanced around and laughed out loud. Imagine me, little Shawna Schuh, in a "star wagon," but with no one to show off to. I checked out the furnishings, the microwave, VCR and television. After a few minutes, I became uncomfortable, so out I went to the craft services area where everyone who wasn't anyone hung out. I felt better there.

When they came and got me for makeup, I was stuffing M&Ms into my mouth and feeling ridiculous, trying to act confident. The PA came up to me with his walkie-talkie and said, "Miss Schuh, they'll take you in makeup now." I giggled and thanked him.

Star treatment was quite an experience, but I knew that next time I could be back to day player, or whatever. The best part of the entertainment business is its unpredictability. The worst part of the entertainment business is its unpredictability. I decided to enjoy the experience as much as I could. There are so many variables with acting that you can never let your guard down or lose sight of why you are there and what you're supposed to be doing.

Films are photographed out of sequence and, as a result, you have to be alert to your evolution as a character and keep your wits about you. This isn't as easy as it sounds when your costar is Gary Busey. If you don't know his name you would certainly know his face if you saw it. Gary has been in many films, most of them B-movie stuff, but he was brilliant as the star of *The Buddy Holly Story,* and he played the tough second banana in the first *Lethal Weapon.* He is also known for being a wild man, doing drugs and getting into motorcycle accidents.

So here we were, Little Miss Scared-Out-of-Her-Wits and the tough guy. I knew I would need to use every shred of confidence I possessed. The first day on the set, the director introduced me to Gary Busey. He completely snubbed me. The director tried again, "Gary, this is Shawna, she plays Marianne." The director had his arm across my shoulders. "She's your sister-in-law," he said, "the one you're in half the film with."

"Yeah right…Hi." came the gruff reply.

I was unimpressed. Okay, so my part wasn't that big, but it was pivotal, and I had been selected instead of a lot of other women. The director rolled his eyes at me in mock disgust and I knew I wasn't in Helvetia, Oregon, anymore.

Making movies is a long, tedious process and the real talent is behind the cameras doing the planning, the arranging, the directing, and making the pieces fit together. I'm not discounting the part of the actor at all. Without the actors there would be no films, and I love films with wild abandon, but there is a lot that needs to be done while you are waiting for your next scene. I found all the delays frustrating, because I am a doer and a mover. I wanted to get going or move on. The whole filmmaking process became a tiresome bore, probably because I didn't have the temperament for it.

I never once felt as though I had found what I was supposed to do or be. I didn't arrive on the set and say to myself, "This is it; this is what I want to do with my life." I thought that maybe I would, I had dreamed of being in movies, of seeing myself on the screen, but after performing a couple of times in films, I had no burning desire to do it again. Especially if I had to revert to day-player status and the honey-wagon dressing room.

The big scene I had with Gary Busey was when I arrived at the house after my husband died and Gary confronted me about whether or not my husband, his brother, was dealing dope, because he had found some in his brother's belongings. My character was confused and angry that he would even consider the possibility.

"Marianne, I need to ask you a question," Gary said in a somber, serious tone.

I acquired a questioning look. "Of course," I replied on cue.

"Marianne," slight pause for effect, "was Stony dealing dope?" He gazes deep into my eyes to determine what I might or might not know.

I looked back at him in amazement and bewilderment. "No, of course not," I shook my head in denial.

Gary grabbed me fiercely by the shoulders. "Then why did he have a kilo of pot in his safe?" he said, accusing now, intense and demanding.

I was confused and at a loss for words until it dawned on me what was taking place here. "No, no, he would never..." I stopped. This was a big moment.

"How could you think that?" I demanded. I was hurt and insulted, as I was supposed to be. I flung his hands away from me. "You, of all people! For God's sake, Jim (his character's name), he was your brother!" I spat this last line out between clenched teeth and stormed into the house.

We rehearsed the long shot and went over the blocking and movements. I was into it and enjoying that we were finally working. Gary was intense, he was always intense. The long shot went well, we did about three or four takes. It came time for the closeups and they began to tear down and set up for Gary's closeup. They always do the star's closeup first, no matter which is more convenient. It's a sign of respect for the top billed actor. Just as they were beginning to move the camera, Gary stopped the director. "Do Shawna's closeup first," he suggested, much to the surprise of the entire crew, the director and me. I gulped. He was showing me respect.

I thought about when he had snubbed me that first day, and how he had behaved during the shoot thus far, and how I had decided that this film business wasn't for me. I smiled and thanked him. There are good deeds from all kinds of people happening every day in every place in the world. I was glad I was standing right there, right then, enjoying my hard-won part and knowing that I had done well. It was a success in many ways, even if not the way I had imagined.

Pickup #42: Embrace unpredictability.

From where you work to what you do, embrace unpre-dictability and you will have more fun and be happier in the long run. I never knew where or when my next job would come and that was both frustrating and the best part. Being on the edge and not secure keeps you light on your feet and ready for anything.

Pickup #43: Know what you don't want.

I really thought I wanted to act until I actually got to work on film sets. The question is, did I fail because I was wrong in my assumptions? I don't think so. I believe learning what you don't want is equally as important as finding what you do want. Sometimes going after a job or career you always envisioned as ideal is the only way to really put doubt behind you.

I met a woman once who had spent over nine years in school to become a veterinarian. After she worked at it for awhile she determined she didn't want to work with sick animals that owners refused to pay to heal, so she left that career to search for something else. I admire her courage, because it takes gumption to change course and be happy rather than continue to pursue something you once thought you wanted.

Pickup #44: Build respect by your actions.

James Garner was highly respected on set because he was a total professional at all times. He knew his craft and paid attention. He didn't have to demand anything because he had built his reputation by his actions. He is an excellent example of what can happen when you are the real deal, when you do as you say, when you are prepared and professional. Having a goal to gain respect and build a stellar reputation is a wonderful motivator and a top-notch way to live.

Pickup #45: Expect the best.

During my time of exploring the entertainment field in several forms, I listened to and believed a lot of fabulous motivators. Zig Ziglar implored me to "expect the best" and I took his advice. It turned out that I was less disappointed with people when I wore my expectations like a coat and they protected me from negative responses and people. I still expect people to like me, treat me well, and be open and honest. I think most people are. I shouldn't have been surprised that day Gary Busey let me have my closeup first; I didn't know what to expect, but I did expect the best.

So...

Embrace unpredictability.

Know what you don't want.

Build respect by your actions.

Expect the best.

13

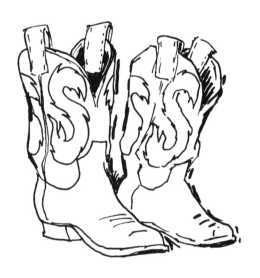

Be Grateful

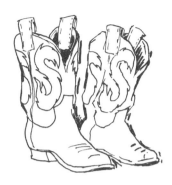

Be Grateful

You can give without loving, but you cannot love without giving.

— Amy Carmichael

When I drove up to the barn, the truck and trailer were parked directly in front of the entrance to the arena. The outside lights were ablaze and, as I pulled up to a stop, I could see Don just inside the arena brushing the new horse's tail.

My first impression of the scene was a good one. Don seemed happy and the horse, even with his hind end to me, seemed content. Also, it was amazing how similar the two appeared. There was Don with his deep red hair showing some gray on the temples and the top, and his massive shoulders and masculine build. The gelding, standing next to Don, was a match in color to Don's red hair, with whiteness sprinkled throughout the red. Four white socks, a white face and one blue eye completed the gelding's identity. The pair, man and horse, were a compatible match, both well built and showing lines of strength.

"So this is him," I said as I made my way in high heels through the damp sand in the aisleway over to the dry sand of the arena. I patted the horse's neck and waited for a reaction. Some horses are social and some are not. This one turned and gave me a sniff. Standing there in my business suit with a raincoat over it and my pantyhose and pumps, I probably smelled funny to him as I rubbed him on the side of his face and he rubbed back against my hand.

"He is so great to ride!" Don said enthusiastically as he continued to work on the horse's tail. "He's like sitting in a rocking chair!" It was obvious that Don was excited and happy to have this new addition to our already healthy family. The gelding made a total of three horses in the barn along with our more than forty head of cattle, four dogs, two cats and two pigs.

"So do you like him?" I said to Don, stating the obvious.

"I really do."

"I've been thinking about this horse," I said. "I think you were supposed to have him, and that he's not like any other horse you might have gotten."

"I've been thinking the same thing myself," Don said, encouraged.

"It's really terrible that Pete had to sell him and I'm sorry about the situation, but maybe it's another example of how God works." I let my words hang in the air of the arena like the mist from our breath.

Don was listening and seemed receptive to the direction I was heading so I continued, "Because Pete wanted you to have him, and because you respect Pete so much, maybe this horse can be the thing that helps you to get back some of the passion you've lost about horses. I think it's a pretty important responsibility, don't you?" I glanced at

Don as he worked methodically with the brush to smooth out the tangles in the horse's tail.

"I've done a lot of thinking ever since Patty called," he started. Patty was Pete's wife of many years and they were a team, just like Don and I. When we first decided to run team pennings at our arena, we called Pete and Patty to let them know we were starting and we talked with them about everything.

Pete and Patty had been running successful pennings for years and were well known all across the country and we didn't want our ambitions to conflict with them in any way. Because of the kind of people they were, they welcomed us in with open arms and hearts and helped us a lot at the beginning with advice and suggestions.

"It's a terrible thing about Pete's cancer," Don continued. "I was so moved that they thought I should have Pete's horse that I almost can't explain my feelings." Don never stopped brushing the tail of the horse.

"I can't help Pete with his cancer," Don added matter-of-factly, "but I can honor him by caring for something he loved." He stopped brushing for a moment. "That's why I'm going to call the horse PT." He looked at me and smiled. "PT, for Pete's Troy. I think God was at work here too."

I smiled at Don and reached up to stroke under PT's mane, which was thick and heavy and had that wonderful coarseness to it. This horse was a social one and had a gentleness to him. I didn't say anything because the moment was pretty special. We were sharing an instant that would be suspended in my mind for many years to come. The height and size of our arena made it appear cathedral-like to me at that moment, and the air was crisp and fresh. The animal that stood between us had given his former owner much love and happiness and now this was spreading to us. There is a pattern to things in the country. The seasons change; life, love and death happen with reasonable certainty, and the predictability is comforting. Pete and Patty were a good, decent couple who had helped and inspired hundreds of people, including Don and me. The example of their marriage was a good one to follow and even in a time of sorrow and pain they continued to spread love to others.

I felt humbled to be a part of their pattern so I wound my arms around PT's massive neck and buried my face in the corner of his jaw. "I'm glad you got him," I mumbled to Don. "He's a wonderful gift." I said a silent prayer that Pete and Patty would understand that they had made the right decision in selling him to us. PT would stand as a testament to their thoughtfulness, strength and love.

In that moment, as I embraced PT, I understood deeply that each of us has a responsibility to care for the gifts we are given. A horse is one example, but trust is another, along with love and faithfulness. We are as fragile as the leaves of the trees that grow and mature and give shade and beauty, but then are whisked away by the breeze that floats in the air and are dropped on the earth where we will break down and become part of the soil that helps the next leaves to grow.

It's not a sad thing to think that you are spreading yourself out to the fullest you can reach as you grow. That's part of the mysterious, marvelous plan. So are the many strong winds that tug and pull at a leaf anchored on the tree that is its family. We are born to cling and resist and eventually to let go, having learned, if we are lucky, that we are part of the seasons. Sometimes the wind that blows is strong and powerful and sometimes it's soft and gentle, but always it blows. In the blowing we are inspired and strengthened again and again.

I looked up at Don and smiled. "I love you," I told him.

"I love you too," he said as he led PT to his stall. I waited at the gate for Don as he turned the lights out one by one. Then we stood for a moment in the darkness until it began to rain.

Pickup #46: Be grateful for all of your gifts.

Other people have been very gracious to me in my life, which is one form of a gift. I have talents and abilities that God has given me, which are other gifts. I know that life and being able to live it in my own way is an incredible gift. Consider all the things you are, and have, and can do, and you will always feel inspired.

Pickup #47: Take responsibility.

In analyzing all the unique and satisfying gifts I've been given it strikes me that I am now responsible for using them, caring for them, loving them and giving myself. This is a tremendous way to get going. It's my job to move on, to grow and give and love and be. I'm totally responsible for my life so I had better keep going.

Pickup #48: Be like a tree.

Have your feet firmly planted and keep reaching, stretching and growing towards the sky. We are like leaves that stretch and reach and hang on during bad weather and good. We are part of a bigger picture and we will ccase to be someday. It's reassuring to know that by our living we have made it better for those who will come behind us. Grow as high as you can, be as big as you want, stretch for miles and miles; the wind won't knock you down, it will only make you stronger.

So...

Be grateful for all of your gifts.

Take responsibility.

Be like a tree.

14

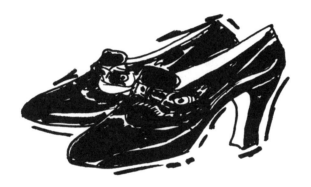

Learn to Give

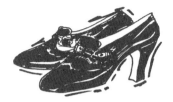

Learn to Give

The more you learn what to do with yourself, and the more you do for others, the more you will learn to enjoy the abundant life.

—William J. H. Boetcker

The room was packed with people. The atmosphere was energetic and fun. About 250 people dressed in business suits were listening to the CEO's presentation. My body was sweating and I could feel perspiration trickle down my sides. I was up next. My mind was racing a mile a minute with all the thoughts one has seconds before speaking to a roomful of highly professional individuals who want good information presented in an uplifting way. Total panic.

My speech was scheduled for 10:30 in the morning; I had arrived in Salt Lake City at 9:08 A.M. The meeting planner, who had picked me up at the airport, had driven at breakneck speed. Talk about cutting it close! I had tried to fly in the day before, but my connecting flight in Seattle had been canceled. Because it was the beginning of spring break in Washington, the alternate flights filled up before

I could exchange my ticket. I had spent the night in a hotel room in Seattle while my overnight bag spent the night in Salt Lake City. I had started the morning without my personal hygiene stuff and brushed my teeth with an emergency kit provided by the airline. I wasn't a mess but I wasn't at my best either.

I shifted my mind onto the audience members to divert my attention from the uneasy feeling in my stomach. I saw well-dressed men and women who were involved in the service business. They were an experienced group, who had heard numerous speakers at their annual conventions. I searched the crowd for someone to connect with, someone who looked like they enjoyed having fun. I spotted some likely candidates sitting to the right of the stage. They looked bright and happy, and I decided I would engage them when it came my time to speak.

As the company's president droned on for several more minutes, I convinced myself that everyone would love me when I spoke, because I would love them when I got up there. Give it all you've got! I said silently as the president began my introduction. I floated up to the stage without touching the ground and found myself in front of 250 questioning faces. I began, "Last summer I was getting ready for a very important presentation to a highly conservative, international accounting firm." All eyes were on me and I had their attention, so far so good.

"I was behind and feeling overwhelmed." A few nods from the audience told me they had been there themselves. "So I had the overheads and handouts professionally prepared." I was doing well, following the story, people seemed interested.

"But when I pulled the handouts out of the package in preparation for the next day's presentation, I realized that the name of this highly conservative, internationally renowned accounting firm, Howard Schultz & Associates, had been printed as 'Howard Stern & Associates.'" It took a moment of realization and then they laughed! Now they knew we were in for some fun!

As I spoke, and shared, and bared my soul, I know I didn't always look pretty—my stories are sometimes ugly, sad or unflattering to me—but I knew that I spoke truthfully and honestly. I only shared what I felt would make a point or make a difference. I was alive! I was in a state of total giving. I finally felt like I had found "home."

I spent the first thirty-five years of my life learning lessons, working toward becoming someone, anyone. But I was always dissatisfied with what I had after I attained it. My life has been a series of trials and errors, open opportunities and some painful lessons. I did what I wanted most of the time and didn't find what I was looking for. Then I discovered that the things that happened to me and the lessons I learned so early in my life and career were all meant to bring me to this point, this sharing of my experiences and knowledge with other people who are searching just like me.

I spent years looking for a way to make myself a star, the focal point. Everything was always about me. The more research I did, the more I learned, the more I realized that a pursuit so narrow would never bring me happiness and joy. My talents are varied and I worked hard to be the best performer I could so that people would want to watch me. It was only when I began to speak to others that I realized that my talent was sharing myself and my experiences to help others.

The minute I quit asking myself about "me" and began to concentrate on what I could give to my audiences, my life changed and I knew exactly what I was supposed to do and be. I am a conduit for God. I am a vessel to be used to promote thinking, confidence and communication. I am only a lens that does its best work when focused outside myself.

Knowing these things has given me a better understanding of how important the journey to this place has been. Had I not tried everything I ever thought I wanted, I wouldn't know how false my assumptions were. But I did try everything, and found all of it lacking. When I stood on the stage and gave from my heart, I knew all of the lessons up to this point had been worth it.

I speak for a living now. I also help organizations and individuals to communicate better. I do it by actively listening, by caring more about successful outcomes for them than successful compliments for me. I have learned that others' successes ensure my own.

I haven't quit learning. I go to school, attend seminars, read books constantly and ask mega-numbers of questions of anyone who will answer. Events still happen that I don't like, but woven into each lesson is the realization that my experience might somehow help someone else, which makes the lessons even more valuable to me. I am growing as I continue to give.

The presentation was well received. Peggy, a meeting planner and a wonderful woman, drove me to the airport. I hadn't seen her during my presentation, so when she complimented me, I was a bit surprised. "Did you hear me speak then?" I asked to make sure I hadn't misheard her. "I didn't see you there."

"I heard enough to know," she said as we drove into the afternoon sun.

"Know what?" I was intrigued.

"Some speakers speak to glorify themselves and some speak for the audience." She paused. "It's obvious you speak to serve."

I smiled, satisfied that my life lessons had been worth learning.

Pickup #49: Give to others.

I found my calling by following my heart and doing all the things I ever thought I wanted. Each time I attained something I had strived for I was dissatisfied and unfulfilled until I turned my attention to others. Jesus washed his disciples' feet; how can I live my life any differently?

Pickup #50: Love people.

I don't worry about people liking me because I believe they know I am loving them. I truly have only one thing in my heart and mind in my work and that's how I can share in such a way that I can make their journey easier or better. What do people need to hear right now that they have forgotten, or that they needed an illustration to see? As I use my mind and talent I am always given the answer and I never stop loving. Love people and you will have more energy than you know what to do with.

Pickup #51: Trust God.

The fifty pickups before this were all action steps—things to do, try, think. I know they work because they have worked for me and others. But action without belief is as futile as baking a cake without flour. It won't come out right and will be nearly impossible to swallow. If you aren't certain there is a God, pick up and begin reading the Bible, or the Koran or any of the spiritual literature available. You

will find answers only when you seek them. Trust that all
the answers are there. They are.

So...

Give to others.

Love people.

Trust God.

51 Pickups

Pickup #1:   Follow your own dream.

Pickup #2:   Dance to the music that moves you.

Pickup #3:   Stay humble.

Pickup #4:   Find the one who needs you.

Pickup #5:   Ask for help when you need it.

Pickup #6:   Do all you can with what you have.

Pickup #7:   Be proud of your efforts.

Pickup #8:   Believe and it will happen for you.

Pickup #9:   Be open to wonder.

Pickup #10: Design some traditions to give stability to your life.

Pickup #11: Trust your heart to give you the answers.

Pickup #12: Find someone who will tell you the truth.

Pickup #13: Be open to learning all things even when they appear unpleasant at first.

Pickup #14: Recognize that you are not stupid if you don't know something.

Pickup #15:   Have a good cry when you're disappointed.

Pickup #16:   Do the right thing no matter what the circumstances.

Pickup #17:   Always talk "with" people.

Pickup #18:   Open the drapes and let the sun in!

Pickup #19:   Forgive and move on.

Pickup #20:   Don't give up until you get what you want.

Pickup #21:   Try things even when you're scared of them.

Pickup #22:   Learning to stop is as important as learning to go.

Pickup #23:   Take the risk so you never have to wonder

Pickup #24:   When risks don't work out, don't make the same mistake twice.

Pickup #25:   Keep on asking yourself, "Is this all there is?"

Pickup #26:   Be curious.

Pickup #27:   Have a system in place for getting through upsetting times.

Pickup #28:   Pick the right time to suggest changes and ideas.

Pickup #29:   Learn to be alone.

Pickup #30: Pull yourself up and face the music.

Pickup #31: Know that opportunities are endless.

Pickup #32: Stay focused.

Pickup #33: Ask for what you want.

Pickup #34: Keep your faith.

Pickup #35: Keep going even when you're discouraged.

Pickup #36: Do your best work, regardless of your position.

Pickup #37: Be overprepared for everything.

Pickup #38: Dress up for others.

Pickup #39: Stick with your instincts.

Pickup #40: Try new things.

Pickup #41: Be ready for the unexpected.

Pickup #42: Embrace unpredictability.

Pickup #43: Know what you don't want.

Pickup #44: Build respect by your actions.

Pickup #45: Expect the best.

Pickup #46: Be grateful for all of your gifts.

Pickup #47: Take responsibility.

Pickup #48: Be like a tree.

Pickup #49: Give to others.

Pickup #50: Love people.

Pickup #51: Trust God.

Shawna Schuh tells stories, laughs, cries, shares information and generally has a ton of fun as she delivers to her audiences comical content that makes a difference. Open your next event with a Kick from the Schuh! Shawna is an entertaining and energetic keynoter who brings soul to any situation!

Contact Shawna at:

Shawna Schuh
24241 Highway 47
Gaston, Oregon 97119

Toll-free: 1-877-4Shawna
Fax: 503-662-4381
e-mail: Shawna@Shu-Biz.com

Note: Shawna would love to hear from you
about ways that you
Pick Up Your Get-Up-and-Go!

Shawna Schuh is the creator of **Social-Graces.com,** a **Daily Dose of Graciousness** that comes to you every day by e-mail to help you put your best foot forward. Building character is like building a muscle. **Daily Doses of Graciousness** let you build your manners muscle without the sweat but with many benefits. We welcome you to visit our web site and learn how our **Daily Doses of Graciousness** can benefit you!

www.Social-Graces.com

To order additional copies of

51 Ways to Pick Up
Your Get-Up-and-Go

Book: $14.95   Shipping/Handling: $3.50

Contact: **BookPartners, Inc.**
P.O. Box 922, Wilsonville, OR 97070
Fax: 503-682-8684
Phone: 503-682-9821
Phone: 1-800-895-7323